ISSUES IN
COMMUNITY PSYCHOLOGY
AND PREVENTIVE
MENTAL HEALTH

COMMUNITY MENTAL HEALTH SERIES

Sheldon R. Roen, Ed.

Research Contributions from Psychology to Community Mental Health / Edited by Jerry W. Carter, Jr.

From Dependency to Dignity: Individual and Social Consequences of a Neighborhood House / Louis A. Zurcher and Alvin E. Green with Edward Johnson and Samuel Patton

Coordinate Index Reference Guide to Community Mental Health / Stuart E. Golann

Mental Health and the Community: Problems, Programs, and Strategies / Edited by Milton F. Shore and Fortune V. Mannino

Children of Mentally Ill Parents: Problems in Child Care / Elizabeth P. Rice, Miriam C. Ekdahl, and Leo Miller

Mental Health Related Activities of Companies and Unions: A Survey Based on the Metropolitan Chicago Area / Elizabeth J. Slotkin, Leo Levy, Edwin Wetmore, and Ferdinand N. Runk

Brief Therapies / Edited by Harvey H. Barten

Issues in Community Psychology and Preventive Mental Health / Division 27 of the American Psychological Association

The Mental Health Team in the Schools / Margaret Morgan Lawrence

Challenge to Community Psychiatry: A Dialogue Between two Faculties / Edited by Archie R. Foley

The Indigenous Nonprofessional: A Strategy of Change in Community Action and Community Mental Health Programs / Robert Reiff and Frank Riessman, Second Edition

Controversies in Community Mental Health / Harry Gottesfeld

The Therapeutic Community: A Source Book of Readings / Edited by Jean J. Rossi and William J. Filstead

ISSUES IN COMMUNITY PSYCHOLOGY AND PREVENTIVE MENTAL HEALTH

by the TASK FORCE ON COMMUNITY MENTAL HEALTH,
DIVISION 27 OF THE
AMERICAN PSYCHOLOGICAL ASSOCIATION,

John C. Glidewell, Ph.D., Chairman

Book Editor: **Gershen Rosenblum, Ph.D.**, *Region V Mental Health Administrator, Department of Mental Health, Dedham, Massachusetts*

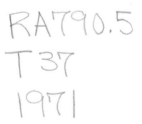
Behavioral Publications Inc. · New York

Library of Congress Catalog Card Number 75-140047
Standard Book Number 87705-022-8
Copyright © 1971 by the Task Force on Community Mental Health,
Division 27 of the American Psychological Association

BEHAVIORAL PUBLICATIONS, INC.,
2852 Broadway—Morningside Heights
New York, New York 10025

Printed in the United States of America

DIVISION 27 OF THE AMERICAN PSYCHOLOGICAL ASSOCIATION

THE TASK FORCE ON COMMUNITY MENTAL HEALTH

Committee Members*

John C. Glidewell, Ph.D., *Chairman*
Mortimer Brown, Ph.D., *Co-Chairman*

Bernard L. Bloom, Ph.D., *University of Colorado, Boulder, Colorado*
Louis D. Cohen, Ph.D., *University of Florida, Gainesville, Florida*
Herbert Dörken, Ph.D., *Chief, Bureau of Research, California Department of Mental Hygiene, Los Angeles, California*
Wilbert Edgerton, Ph.D., *Department of Psychology, The School of Medicine, University of North Carolina, Chapel Hill, North Carolina*
Ira Iscoe, Ph.D., *Department of Psychology, University of Texas, Austin, Texas*
James G. Kelly, Ph.D., *Department of Psychology and Institute for Social Research, University of Michigan, Ann Arbor, Michigan*
Robert Reiff, Ph.D., *Albert Einstein College of Medicine, New York, New York*

*We acknowledge the assistance of Ija Korner, Ph.D. and Gershen Rosenblum, Ph.D. in the compilation, editing, and indexing of this book.

Contents

Preface
    D. C. Klein ix
Introduction
    I. N. Korner xi

1: **Strategies for the Prevention of Mental Disorders**
    B. L. Bloom 1

2: **Professional and Subprofessional Training in Community Mental Health as an Aspect of Community Psychology**
    I. Iscoe 21

3: **Community Psychology and Public Policy**
    R. Reiff 33

4: **Health and Disease: Observations on Strategies for Community Psychology**
    L. D. Cohen 55

5: **A Dimensional Strategy for Community Focused Mental Health Services**
    H. Dörken 75

6: **Evaluation in Community Mental Health**
    J. W. Edgerton 89

7: **The Quest for Valid Preventive Interventions**
    J. G. Kelly 109

8: Priorities for Psychologists in Community Mental Health
     J. Glidewell 141

Index 155

Preface

Five years after its emergence as a denotable emphasis within psychology, the field of community psychology continues its search for a consensual identity. The present volume is a major contribution to that search. Rather than placing the field within the perspective of the mental health movement, it seeks to forge a distinctive statement of a community psychology focus for the mental health enterprise itself. The book is a product of the efforts of a task force requested by the Division of Community Psychology to look into the mental health field from the community psychologist's perspective.

It is no accident that this early statement of identity for community psychology emerges in relationship to mental health. As the report of the Swampscott Conference (Boston University and South Shore Mental Health Center, Quincy, Mass., 1966) shows, the very creation of a converging community emphasis within psychology occurred as a result of psychologists' exposure to community dynamics through their participation in the mental health movement. Even today most community psychologists are clinically trained individuals who have earned their community spurs within community mental health programs. With a few notable exceptions, the training programs in community psychology are subspecialties within graduate programs in clinical psychology, although there are those who look forward to training that will encompass other subspecialties such as social and developmental.

For a time it appeared that community psychology would become the umbrella area within the profession, with community mental health becoming simply a sub-focus. Now, however, it seems more useful to view community psychology and community mental health as two separate, although overlapping, areas for study and practice. Community mental health is more than community psychology—it is concerned with genetics, physical as well as psychological trauma, biochemical concomitants of emotional disorders, and a whole host of factors which are not subsumed under community psychology. The latter field, in turn, draws increasingly from education, physical and social planning, a variety of social movements, social anthropology, and many other areas of inquiry and practice not usually considered to be central to the mental health focus.

The book may signal the coming of age of community psychology. It views community mental health as a co-equal. It draws on the community psychologist's strength as participant-conceptualizer to develop the thesis that primary prevention is not only *a possible emphasis* within mental health, it is *the only defensible emphasis* if the field is to escape from the impossible task of trying to prevent emotional disorders by treating them wholesale once they have manifested themselves. For the community psychologist, the task appears to be the painstaking one of increasing our understanding of man-in-environment; that is, the interactions whereby the community shapes the development of individuals, introduces stress into their lives, and mediates the ways in which the emotional hazards of living are dealt with for better or worse. One key to primary prevention in mental health, the community psychologist holds, is the community itself. As we shape the community towards meeting the needs of individuals for safety, security, and personal significance throughout the life cycle, we become truly engaged with mental *health* rather than mental *disorder*.

Donald C. Klein, Ph.D.
Past President, Division 27,
American Psychological Association

[1] Boston University and South Shore Mental Health Center, Quincy, Mass., "A Report of the Boston Conference on the Education of Psychologists for Community Mental Health," *Community Psychology*, 1966.

Introduction

I. N. Korner

The reports submitted form a whole.

The "Final Report" by Glidewell summarizes what representatives of the field observe, think about, criticize, and convert into abstractions and generalizations. The "Final Report" describes the status of the field and charts some of its future. The "Support Papers" subtly blend into the substance of the "Final Report".

The "Support Papers" demonstrate the function of the academic and administrative layer in psychology. Academicians absorb from their students and their own work in professional situations knowledge of the success and failure of their endeavors. They respond with their academic and social reflexes; they criticize, reformulate, reconceptualize. The papers by Bloom, Iscoe, Reiff, and Cohen fall into this category.

Administrators of programs hear from the population they serve. If dissatisfaction is voiced, if objective findings bear out that programs do not achieve what they are designed for, the theories underlying the practice are in need of changing. The paper by H. Dörken is characteristic of this trend.

True to their vocations, psychologists tend toward experimental screening of their activities. There is an additional element which forces the psychologists in the community mental health field to greater use of the research tool. The social institutions providing the financial resources for mental and community health endeavors have learned to ask the right questions, to demand an accounting. They ask: How well do you spend the dollars allotted? Do you deliver what a specific program promises at a reasonable cost? The paper by Edgerton deals with the general issue of research and mental and community health practice. Subsequently, only do research theoreticians and research specialists develop methods, first in theory and later in trial and error practice, to provide the requested evaluative answers. The paper by Kelly describes this process.

The "Final Report" is more than the sum of the support papers—it is the expression of Division 27 today. It should be referred to as provisional-final, keeping in focus this division's concern with the changing needs of society and the efforts of its members to be part of the change.

1: Strategies for the Prevention of Mental Disorders

Bernard L. Bloom

The great task still before us in the field of community mental health is primary prevention, that is, the reduction of the incidence of those kinds of maladaptive behaviors which are designated as mental disorders. That this task still lies before us is testimony to the failure of the current community health movement to heed the words of John F. Kennedy who in his historic presidential message of February 5, 1963, stated that "First, we must seek out the causes of mental illness and of mental retardation and eradicate them . . . For prevention is far more desirable for all concerned. It is far more economical and it is far more likely to be successful. Prevention will require both selected specific programs directed especially at known causes, and the general strengthening of our fundamental community, social welfare, and educational programs which can do much to eliminate or correct the harsh environmental conditions which often are associated with mental retardation and mental illness"[11] Contrary to the Presidential assertion that in the new comprehensive community mental health centers, prevention as well as treatment would be a major activity, staff resources are almost totally deployed thus far in the provision of relatively traditional services.[16]

Lest one think that the interest in the prevention of mental disorders is new, it is well to remember the words of Adolf Meyer written more than fifty years ago: "Communities have to learn what they *produce* in the way of mental problems and waste of human opportunities, and with such knowledge they will rise from mere charity and mere mending, or hasty propaganda, to well-balanced early care, prevention and general gain of health."[5] Add to this the words of Harry Stack Sullivan written in 1931: "Either you believe that mental disorders are acts of God, predestined, inexorably fixed, arising from a constitutional

or some other irremediable substratum, the victims of which are to be
helped through an innocuous life to a more or less euthanasic
exit . . . *or* you believe that mental disorder is largely preventable and
somewhat remediable by control of psycho-sociological factors."[5]
These earlier calls to preventive action were echoed in the 1963
Presidential Message to the United States Congress on the subject of
mental illness and mental retardation and together outline a value, a
theory, and a program. The value is that these behaviors often labeled
as mental disorders are undesirable and should be eliminated. The
theory asserts that causes of a significant proportion of mental
disorders lie in man's society, in the harsh environmental and
psychosociological conditions under which many of us live. The
program is to identify these environmental community conditions and
change them with the hope, strengthened by good evaluative research,
that the subsequent incidence of maladaptive behaviors will be
significantly reduced.

Instead of being oriented around this hopeful and exciting preventive
focus, the community mental health center movement is attempting to
provide a somewhat expanded and better integrated array of treatment
services in the community, but as Smith has recently indicated, these
treatment services don't reach those who need help most, these
expended programs cannot conceivably be staffed, and the potential of
the community for bad or good isn't recognized. With regard to this
latter point, he wrote: "We are not dealing with isolated disease
processes, but with vicious circles of human misery and ineffectiveness,
with patterns of self-defeating behavior that are hard to break because
they are embedded in the very texture of people's lives. We need to
invest more in working on the social contexts in which troubled people
are involved, and to count less upon the effectiveness of the isolated
therapeutic hour."[20]

It is most appropriate to view preventive activities as the great hope.
A brief review of medical history will demonstrate that prevention has
been significantly more powerful than treatment in reducing the
prevalence of most diseases. This is true for both the infectious as well
as the nutritional diseases and should be equally true for the vast
reservoirs of the chronic conditions among which will be found mental

disorders. Long before the advent and acceptance of germ theory with its implications of specific diagnosis and disease-specific treatment, the sanitarians and humanitarians had combined to indict odors and odor-producing accumulation of filth as the cause of all disease and to propose a massive clean-up campaign and sewage disposal system as a disease preventive. The emphasis on cleanliness and on the eradication of miasmas or noxious odors had enormous consequences for disease incidence. By 1800, maternal mortality had dropped to one-seventh of its level of 1750. Typhoid fever, yellow fever, tuberculosis, typhus, cholera and infant mortality all were sharply reduced independently of germ theory. Indeed, it is not generally known but the nursing profession was started by Florence Nightingale during the time of the Crimean War as a protest against germ theory. The current community mental health movement, with its occasional emphasis upon the removal of existing accumulations of psychic sewage and its efforts to prevent its further accumulation is a logical and most appropriate descendant of the sanitary awakening of more than a century ago, and we have much to learn from the miasmatists of old. (See Bloom, 1965.)

It is probably idle to speculate about the reasons for the failure of the community mental health movement to involve itself properly with preventive programs, although once psychiatry rejoined the so-called "mainstream of medicine" it should not have surprised anyone that preventive services in mental health would have had the same low priority as preventive medicine in general. Rather, we need to ask a series of questions regarding primary prevention. What are the issues? What are the strategies? What kinds of research programs need to be undertaken to form the empirical foundation for these strategies?

Issues and Strategies in Primary Prevention

The fundamental issue in primary prevention may very well be whether our society will permit mental disorders to be prevented. Significant modification of social conditions under which many people live will be exceedingly costly in money and in stress upon many segments of professional and lay society. There is some evidence that the

most disadvantaged groups in our society may not trust the mental
health enterprise (see Keniston, 1968). We may discover that the
motive of preventing mental disorders may conflict with other motives,
for example, the wish for privacy and anonymity and the strong desire
to be left alone. At the organizational level we must recognize that our
society and its social institutions are based upon the assumption that
mental disorders will occur, that special facilities for the treatment or
the storage of persons who fail to survive our primary social institutions
need to be constructed and manned. Finally, there may be some
fundamental truth in the commonly held belief that we all need to be
able to identify persons less fortunate and less productive than
ourselves. From this point of view it may be that preventive efforts will
fail because, simply stated, our society needs its mentally ill. Thus to
consider seriously that emotional disorders can be prevented in
significant numbers without requiring some painful adjustments in
societal values, community organization and professional practices may
be quite naive. Successful preventive programs require increased
capacity on the part of our primary institutions, our homes and schools
most particularly, to retain their members instead of ejecting them. At
the same time we need to make courageous changes in our social
agencies and in the ways mental health professionals spend their
working days. Intensive psychotherapy may be useful for the individual
patient but as a major program strategy it is clearly ineffective in
reducing the total amount of community psychopathology.

What strategies are available to the mental health professional
interested in primary prevention? There are obviously two broad
categories, namely increasing man's resistance to stress-inducing psycho-
social forces within the community, on the one hand, and reducing
these stresses on the other hand.

Intervention with the Individual

Increasing man's tolerance of stress and his skill in dealing with it is
already an attractive goal to most mental health professionals. Crises
will occur and if one believes that successful crisis resolutions are

cumulative and can result in increasing emotional well-being, then opportunities for constructive intervention around both normative as well as unanticipated crises can result in a significant reduction in the incidence of emotional disorders. Thus far in the development of points of view regarding primary prevention techniques applied to the individual, three tactics have been proposed. First, techniques of crisis intervention are being developed based upon the belief that mental health professionals can make a significant community-wide impact if they pick their spots, identifying persons in crisis and intervening briefly at those moments when such persons can be helped to resolve the crisis in a favorable manner. A second tactic has been called anticipatory guidance, that is, the pre-solution of anticipated crises. The most common method utilized thus far has been the group meeting, such as between the clergyman and his engaged parishioners or between the hospital-based medical social worker and a group of new parents. The third tactic is consultation, the process whereby the skilled mental health practitioner assists the public health nurse or school teacher, for example, in meeting the mental health needs of her patients or students. Mental health consultation is based on the premise that this work style will result in the greatest community impact even though the impact from the point of view of the mental health professional is somewhat indirect.

Implicit in these alternative approaches to strengthening man's resistance to psychological stresses, are different views of the process of identifying the recipients of these approaches. One approach has been to aim preventive programs at the total population in a defined geographic area. Programs of water purification and sewage disposal are community-wide in their impact. In the mental health area, efforts at mental health education through the use of the mass media represents an effort to effect a given change in the total community. A second approach to identifying the recipient population for a preventive program is what might be called the milestone program. In this type of program a preventive service is provided to the members of a community when they reach a particular pre-defined point in their life histories, a point usually thought to constitute a normative crisis. A vaccination against smallpox is usually required prior to entrance into

elementary school, although the vaccine is administered at that
particular milestone in a child's life in part because of the ease in
locating the recipient group. In the mental health field, a transition in
public school can be viewed as a developmental crises. The major
intervention program at the Woodlawn Mental Health Center in
Chicago, for example, is with all first grade children in the area this
center serves (see Kellam and Schiff, 1966). Anticipatory guidance
techniques, consultation and crisis intevention can all be employed in
milestone programs.

A third approach has been to identify groups of persons at high risk
of developing that particular set of behaviors which it is hoped the
program will prevent. Because industrial health studies have shown
harmful respiratory effects of certain forms of mining, or the dangers to
the eye when using a grindstone, certain preventive measures
(facemasks or goggles) are usually required. Crisis intervention services
could be instituted for all school-age children upon the death of a
parent or sibling. Consultation could be provided to attorneys with
particular regard to the client petitioning for a divorce on the basis of
evidence liking marital disruption with subsequent psychiatric disability. Anticipatory guidance services could be made available to
workers getting ready to retire, or to housewives whose youngest child
is within a few months of graduating from high school and leaving the
parental home.

While the identification of normative crises can proceed by informal
observation, or by deductions from the analysis of changing role
performance requirements in the developing individual, the identification of high risk groups most usually proceeds from epidemiological
investigations which seek to discover personal characteristics significantly associated with the development of psychiatric disorders.

In viewing these preventive strategies it is useful to keep in mind that,
like water purification or swamp spraying, a program emphasizing
community change can significantly influence the entire community
population. Person-oriented programs are somewhat more limited in
their breadth of influence although, like the smallpox vaccination, they
may be enormously effective. When one takes a broad ecologic view of
mental disorders and their prevention it is easy to become a generalist,

however, and to agree with the argument of Edward Rogers that "general preventive measures directed at the determination and control of the underlying patterns of environmental relationships will prove more efficient and effective in the long run than so-called specific measures."[18]

Intervention in the Community

Modification of community characteristics requires a compassionate empirical analysis of the community and its dimensions, how these impinge on the lives of the persons who live within it, why apparently undesirable characteristics persist, how to enhance the power of growth-inducing community variables, and how to discourage the life styles which seem to be associated with social disequilibrium. In writing about modification of the environment as it applies to youth, Keniston has suggested: "One reason the unrest of youth eludes psychological categories may be psychiatry's stress on the inner world and on those modes of adaptation that Heinz Hartmann has called auto-plastic—efforts at self-change, at insight, at adaptation to the environment. Too little attention has been given to the positive value of alloplastic adaptations, which try to make the world a more livable place, to create new life styles, to change others."[10] We desperately need the humanistically-oriented social scientist to involve himself in the life of the community in order to try to effect community change. And as was indicated earlier, our social agency policies may need to be changed as much as other aspects of the psychosocial environment. A useful concept of which to remind oneself is the notion of the community as a system of identifiable but interdependent parts. The British poet Francis Thompson described this interdependence at a cosmic level when he wrote, "Thou canst not stir a flower without troubling a star."

The community mental health movement appears to be looking beyond its original narrowly defined mandate. Its first phase began with the enactment of the community mental health centers legislation in 1963, and during the early years of the community mental health center movement in the United States the focus was toward returning clinical services to the community. The thrust of the community mental health center program during its initial years encouraged private practitioners to see their patients in community mental health centers, attempted to integrate mental health services with community hospital services, and in most general terms, worked toward improving and expanding direct clinical services and integrating psychiatry with general medicine.

Paralleling this early view of community mental health center program objectives were a series of unusually implicit assumptions regarding community structure. First, it was assumed that community residents could be sorted into those who were disadvantaged and those who were not. Second, it was assumed that some members of the community were caretakers and others were clients of caretakers. Third, it was assumed that the repository of wisdom regarding community mental health needs was the mental health professional and his colleagues in other social agencies. As a consequence of these assumptions, community mental health needs were assessed (see Lemkau, 1967, for example) by asking mental health professionals and other health and welfare workers for their judgments, or by interpolating from current mental health service statistics, taking into account anticipated changes in population characteristics.

This set of assumptions regarding the community and the assessment of its mental health needs has become increasingly untenable. First, as has been mentioned, emphasis on the prevention of mental disorder has increased. It has become clear that while some sources of psychopathology are inside the skin, other sources are within the social systems in which we live and thus that prevention will require more active involvement with the community. Second, if modifications are to be made in these social systems in an effort to prevent or limit the disability associated with psychopathology, some forms of social or political action are going to be required. Third, the area of legitimate concern of the mental health professional has been extended to include interest in factors affecting the entire community, in improving human vitality, and the quality of life. Fourth, with a growing interest in socially generated psychopathology, the related concepts of self-esteem and power have undergone a significant renaissance. Ryan has suggested for example that ". . . self-esteem is to some extent an essential requirement to the very survival of the human organism . . . (and) is partially dependent on the inclusion of a sense of power within the self-concept . . . a mentally healthy person must be able to perceive himself as at least minimally powerful, capable of influencing his environment to his own benefit, and further, . . . this sense of minimal power has to be based on the actual experience, and exercise of power . . . A program of mental health enhancement and emotional disorder prevention, therefore, can meaningfully address itself to the issue of personal and community power."[19] Fifth, even with respect to the provision of direct clinical services it has become increasingly obvious that improvements have to be made in the organization and delivery of these services, in their financing, and in the control of their quality. These improvements may not be made without pressure being exerted by recipients or potential recipients of service, and thus, may not be made without social or political action. Finally, a much more compassionate view of the strengths and weaknesses within the community is appearing. In this view a community is seen not as consisting of givers and takers but as interdependent people *all* of whom have needs which can be met by others and who have contributions to make to others (see Blackman and Goldstein, 1968). In this view, furthermore, *all* members of the community are seen as potentially disadvantaged by poverty and by poor health, to be sure, but also by loss of parents, by job dissatisfactions, by unhappy marriages, and by the lack of a meaningful social role. Many of these sources of disadvantage are independent of socioeconomic affluence.

Yolles has recently written, "There will be no effective national progress in community mental health unless psychiatrists and other core mental health professionals . . . accept their responsibilities as professionals to practice as community leaders and activists as well as clinicians."[21] Thus, a new relationship is required between the mental health professional on the one hand and the community within which he lives and works on the other hand. This relationship focuses on the interdependence of all members of the community, including those members who provide mental health services, and begins with the assumption that wisdom regarding community mental health needs is not limited to mental health professionals, but resides in all members of the community and, in fact, that the mental health professional may have limited knowledge of some of these needs and limited motivation to meet them.

Several principles for developing community mental health related programs can be derived from the foregoing conceptualization of the community.

Principle No. 1 Regardless of where your paycheck comes from, think of yourself as working for the community. Mental health programs in the community should be determined by a process of negotiation involving inputs from all members of the community. The ultimate power for deciding the nature of the community based mental health program should rest with the community, and the mental health professional should work in the community only as long as he feels a sense of congruence between the program desired by the community and his own personal and professional value system.

Principle No. 2 If you want to know about a community's mental health needs, ask them. It is important that in the process of determining community mental health needs one does not limit himself to asking statements of opinion from agency personnel or does not base one's planning solely on extrapolation from present mental health service statistics. There are at least three other techniques which should be mentioned as ways of identifying community needs. First, public hearings can be held whereby any member of the community who has something to say about mental health needs, either his own or those of his family, his friends, or the entire community, can be heard. Second, systematic household surveys can be undertaken in which some sample of persons in the community is identified and interviewed with respect to their impressions of mental health-related needs in the community. Third, psychiatric patients themselves are an invaluable source of information regarding community health-related needs. When a patient is ready to be discharged from psychiatric care, an opportunity presents itself to turn to him for help in exchange for the help he has received. He can be asked to express his own understanding of the needs for mental health-related services in the community. One question that would be particularly useful to ask former psychiatric patients is how the community would have been structured in order for the person not to have developed those kinds of disorganized or disturbing behaviors which resulted in his seeking psychiatric care. Another related question is to ask the patient what things would have had to have happened differently in his own past history in order for him not to have required psychiatric care.

Principle No. 3 As you learn about community mental health-related needs you have the responsibility to tell the community what you are learning. This principle puts the mental health professional in the role of a community educator, an advocate, and a source of moral persuasion. The mental health professional is in an excellent position to learn about situations in the community which need to be corrected, and he should keep in front of the community's consciousness his understanding of these unmet mental health needs and the proposals for action which might be advanced for their solution.

Principle No. 4 Let the community establish its own priorities. When community mental health needs have been identified, it is reasonable to expect that the resources available to the community will not be sufficient to meet all of them. Representatives of the community should play a major role in deciding which needs will be met first and how the limited resources will be deployed among the various identified needs. It is theoretically possible, of course, that needs can conflict with each other, that is, that in the very act of meeting one need, one automatically exacerbates the condition with respect to another need. Out of the identification of these kinds of inconsistencies, programs emerge which capture the concensus of the entire group.

Principle No. 5 You can help the community to decide between various courses of action in its efforts to solve its own problems. This is a special and perhaps unique role for the mental health professional who is acquainted not only with needs and strategies for meeting them in other communities but also with empirical research results. This knowledge can help him advise the community when it tries to make decisions between various courses of action. The mental health professional can identify high risk groups within the community and discuss alternative proposals in dealing with the problems of these groups.

Principle No. 6 In the event that the community being served is so disorganized that representatives of various facets of the community cannot be found, you have the responsibility for assisting in organizing the community. It is crucial in the work of the mental health professional to be certain that he is in good communication with the entire community and its representatives and not merely with selected members of an entrenched power group. The mental health professional should be certain that his own policy-making board is organized in such a way that the members of the board represent all sociocultural groups and socioeconomic levels within the community.

Principle No. 7 You should work toward the equitable distribution of power in the community. While it is difficult to make generalizations about optimal distribution of power, the most equitable way of distributing power appears to be in direct proportion to the population of the various identifiable ethnic subgroups within the community.

To the extent that these principles are carried out, the community becomes involved in its own mental health and emotional vitality, the community increases its power over its own life with a resulting increase in self-esteem, and as a consequence, an increase in emotional robustness and mental health can be anticipated.

It is important to acknowledge that emotional disorders will not be eradicated by assisting members of the community to develop increased self-esteem and increased power over their own lives. Not all psychopathology can be traced to powerlessness or other defects of the social systems within which people live, yet it seems crucial to test the limits of this dynamic view of the community as a system of interdependent human beings and this theory of psychopathology.

The foregoing principles, which have been suggested as being required for the necessary involvement of the total community in developing its mental health programs, are already well accepted with respect to the professional community. This degree of acceptance can be documented by the following quotation from a summary of a conference on Professional Inservice Education. In the following quotation one need only substitute the word "community" for "employee," the phrase "mental health-related activities" for the word "learning," and the phrase "mental health professional" for the word "teacher." "Learning will be most effective when the employees have diagnosed their own needs and formulated their own goals for learning." "Learning will be most effective when engaged in actively by the employees as a process for self-education (or mutual inquiry); the teacher will most effectively help in this process when he perceives himself not as a transmitter of information but as a facilitator and resource to the employee's inquiries." "Employees will feel committed (motivated) to learn to the extent that they are involved in the planning, execution, and evaluation of their own learning experiences."[13]

To place these proposals in a somewhat larger context, the noted Spanish author and diplomat Salvador de Madariaga linked the concepts of power as described above to the judicial concept of freedom. He wrote as follows: "He is free who knows how to keep in his own hands the power to decide at each step the course of his life and who lives in a society which does not block the exercise of that power." It may seem a long jump indeed between the development of preventively-oriented mental health programs in the community and the concept of freedom, yet the principles enunciated above for the identification of community needs are ones which are inextricably interwoven with the concepts of freedom and dignity and these concepts are surely integral parts of the phenomenon known as mental health.

The Role of Epidemiology in Primary Prevention

The research base of primary prevention is rooted in the science and methods of epidemiology. Epidemiology is the study of the distribution and determinants of disease prevalence in man. In studying the distribution of a disease or a disorder, we are involved in the field of descriptive epidemiology. The epidemiologist tries to interpret its distribution so as to identify possible causal factors. When data are collected in such a way as to evaluate these possible causal factors, one speaks of the field of analytic epidemiology. When such analyses lend themselves to trial programs designed to study the power of our causal explanations, we have entered the field of experimental epidemiology.

Thus, descriptive epidemiology shades into demography and human ecology. Analytic epidemiology is related to applied field study research, and experimental epidemiology is sometimes indistinguishable from program evaluation. Epidemiology is thus the basic science of preventive action.

From the time of Hippocrates through the era of the European sanitarians, into the modern era of germ theory and nutritional theory, the epidemiologist has noted that diseases have not been randomly distributed in the population with respect to time characteristics or place characteristics or person characteristics and has sought factors which might be causally related to them by an analysis of these differences in distribution. One after another, the great infectious and nutritional diseases have succumbed to the clinical and environmental research of the epidemiologist, until at the present time it can be asserted that techniques are available for the prevention of virtually every major infectious and nutritional disease. The challenge in the field of the infectious and nutritional diseases at present is in the fact that, in spite of our understanding of the microbiology and physiology of these disorders, they continue to be endemic or epidemic throughout most of the world. The contribution of the epidemiologist has already been made. The fate of these diseases now rests in the hands of the social scientist.

The causal connection between iodine deficiency and exophthalmic goiter is crystal clear, yet in many places in southeast Asia, goiter is not only endemic with its resultant sapping of human productivity, intellect, and life expectancy, but its eradication is struggled against by its very victims because of the belief that without a goiter of optimal size, a Burmese or Loatian or Cambodian woman is not considered a desirable marriage prospect. The goiter in many parts of southeast Asia, much as the female breast in the United States, has taken on a secondary significance unrelated to and often as important as its original function.

Beri-beri, a nutritional disease endemic in the Philippines, can be prevented simply by ceasing to remove the hulls and outer layers of rice before preparing it for eating. Yet an extraordinarily resistant strain of folklore has arisen around this somewhat yellowish outer layer which makes this simple preventive device unpalatable. Typhoid fever, endemic in most Peruvian villages, can be prevented simply by boiling water before using it. Yet again, an entire cultural value system has grown which puts constraints on what and when things may be heated. In the United States, the peculiar custom of breathing in the smoke and fire made by the burning of a carefully cultivated weed resulted last year in the senseless deaths of 45,000 people from lung cancer.

The great unfinished work for the field of epidemiology is in what is generally called the chronic diseases—coronary artery disease, cancer, and the mental disorders, for example. While mental disorders are rarely fatal, as a group they are responsible for more long-lasting misery than any other pathological condition. It is in the search for causal factors regarding these conditions that much of the work of the epidemiologist is now directed.

It is important to be very clear what the epidemiologist means by the concept of cause. If a category of events has a frequency x and another category has a frequency y, the two events, if independent of each other, would be expected to occur in the frequency xy. That is, if one person in a hundred is an orphan by age 18, and one person in a hundred has an emotional disorder, assuming that orphan status and the presence of emotional disorders are unrelated, we would expect that one person in ten thousand would be *both* an orphan by age 18 *and* the victim of an emotional disorder. In order to prove an association between orphan status and emotional disorder, one would have to show first that the frequency of these two characteristics in the same people significantly exceeded the expected rate of one in ten thousand. It is common, of course, for two factors which are statistically associated not to be causally associated.

In order for two factors to be considered causally related, the epidemiologist requires, in addition to statistical association, that there be some consistent time sequence such that the presumed causal event precedes the presumed effect, and that there be a relatively strong association such that should the presumed causal event occur, there is considerable likelihood that the effect will subsequently occur. Thus, to the epidemiologist, Factor A is causally related to Factor B when a change in the frequency of Factor A results or could be presumed to result in a subsequent significant change in the frequency of Factor B. In the case of emotional disorders, then, the epidemiologist is looking for factors reasonably strongly associated with the subsequent development of emotional disorders in the hopes that a program which would reduce the frequency of one or more of these factors would result in the reduced frequency of emotional disorders.

Research thus far in the epidemiology of mental disorders has tended to restrict itself completely to what was earlier called descriptive epidemiology—the study of the distribution of emotional disorders in general or one in particular and the development of hypotheses to account for unusual characteristics of this distribution. Most of this research dates from the now historic work of Faris and Dunham (1939) who more than 25 years ago studied the distribution of schizophrenia in Chicago. More recent studies in this tradition include the work of the Leightons (1963) in Nova Scotia, Langer and his colleagues (1963) in Manhattan, and Klee *et al.* (1967) in Baltimore. These studies are of two types. The demographic studies relate personal characteristics to various rates of mental disorder, and the ecological studies relate neighborhood or other environmental characteristics to mental disorder rates. Both of these types of studies are enormously useful and complementary since they identify high-risk groups of people and high-risk neighborhoods and suggest both people and places with whom and where preventive services can be developed.

Epidemiologists do not feel restricted to studying the distribution or determinants of traditionally viewed disease categories. Using the public health model of a disease as a condition which has causative factors associated with conditions of the host, conditions of the agent, and conditions of the environment, very fruitful studies have been made of the epidemiology of automobile accidents, for example. Host factors, such as driver fatigue or drinking, have been studied. Environmental factors, such as weather conditions, have been identified, and in recent months our attention has been directed to the agent characteristics of the automobile itself in developing causal hypotheses.

With respect to emotional disorders, epidemiologists similarly need not restrict themselves to the study of traditional diagnostic groups. With the general dissatisfaction often expressed regarding the psychiatric classification system of mental disorders, scientists have the opportunity to study the epidemiology of other phenomena—for example, the epidemiology of psychiatric care, or of emotional disorders associated with poverty, or of chronic unemployment, or of powerlessness, or of hallucinations, or of social incompetence, or academic underachievement or any other syndrome, so long as it can be reliably defined. In fact, much can be said for studying the epidemiology of health or of self-actualization, or of symptom recovery. It may well be that some of the most creative work in the next decade undertaken by epidemiologists will be in the study of the distribution and determinants of these newly acknowledged behavior cluster complexes.

Some Special Problems for the Social Scientist

One of the most vexing problems facing anyone interested in the primary prevention of mental disorders lies in the elusive qualities of the phenomena. Not only are an incredible array of behaviors eligible to be labeled as mental disorders, but the process of diagnosis or labeling is, in large measure, a social process, partially independent of characteristics of the identified patient. Since the essential characteristics of the conditions to be prevented have not been determined, or agreed upon, the task of assessing the extent to which such poorly defined disorders have been prevented is understandably difficult.

Community household surveys have repeatedly shown that a high proportion of diagnosable psychotics live in the community and have never been identified by caretaking agencies. What does it mean to attempt to prevent a condition which in the ordinary course of events would never come to the attention of any professional person? What does it mean to try to prevent psychiatric hospitalizations when the standards of eligibility for hospital admission can fluctuate widely depending on administrative policy? The very concept of primary prevention assumes that the condition to be prevented lies within the person, yet the most cursory examination of the process of case identification makes it very clear that the tolerance of the social milieu within which the "patient" functions is often the single most important component of the diagnostic procedure. Behavior of an individual in a warm accepting family-oriented setting will not come to the attention of official community agencies. Identical behavior in a socially isolated individual will often precipitate his admission to a psychiatric facility. As much attention must be paid to changing settings in which persons function and to changing the course of those interpersonal events which now precipitate admission to a mental hospital as to reducing specific kinds of behaviors in the designated patient. If a school system, which formerly ejected troublesome children because they were variously described as disruptive, anxious, poorly motivated, or suffering from behavior disorders, now is able to accept these same children and retain them within the school program, in a sense, the incidence of childhood behavior disorders has been reduced.

The implication of these remarks is that anyone interested in the field of primary prevention must be prepared to answer the question, what specifically are you trying to prevent? Preventive programs may be directed at shoplifting or drug abuse among college students, and mental health professionals might be centrally involved in the program, but many would argue that there is no appreciable evidence that the behaviors being controlled have any relationship to subsequent psychiatric disability. But effectiveness of any preventive effort has to be judged against the answer to this specific question—what are you trying to prevent?

Another emerging problem for psychologists is the fact that concern with the broad social and environmental factors associated with mental disorders is growing throughout the mental health establishment. The Group for the Advancement of Psychiatry, through its Committee on Preventive Psychiatry, for example, has recently prepared an overview of the increasingly important field of community psychiatry.[7] While the major emphasis on community psychiatry is clinical, that is, on the "treatment of patients close to home and family and their minimal social dislocation,"[7] the report emphasizes socioenvironmental forces in psychopathology and the non-clinical, total community orientation of much of the work of the community psychiatrist. An overlapping interest exists between community psychiatry and community psychology, analagous to the overlapping interest of clinical psychiatry and clinical psychology.

No area either of practice or research clearly emerges as the exclusive property of the social scientist. Perhaps our experience of the past two decades in developing effective working relationships between psychiatric and psychological clinicians will be helpful in developing productive modes of collaboration among community-oriented mental health professionals of whatever professional background.

Social scientists need to familiarize themselves with the field of epidemiology, with its methods of approach to the identification of causal factors in mental disorders, however defined. The social scientist functioning in the community mental health setting needs to learn about community structure and its analysis and about techniques for the facilitation of community change. If the behavioral scientist is to make a significant contribution to the mental health of the community, both his research and his applied skills have to be supplemented by the development of new areas of competence. The university, through its regular training program and its involvement in the continuing education of mental health professionals already in the field, has a crucial role to play in this process.

REFERENCES

1. Blackman, S. and Goldstein, K. M., "Some Aspects of a Theory of Community Mental Health", *Community Mental Health Journal*, 1968, 4, 83-90.
2. Bloom, B. L., The Medical Model, Miasma Theory, and Community Mental Health, *Community Mental Health Journal*, 1965, 1, 333-338.
3. Bower, E. M., "Preventive Services for Children," in B. L. Bloom and Dorothy P. Buck (Eds.) *Preventive Services in Mental Health Programs* (Boulder, Colorado: WICHE, 1967).
4. Bower, E. M., "Slicing The Mystique of Prevention With Occam's Razor," *American Journal of Public Health*, 1969, 59, 478-484.
5. Brand, Jeanne L., "The United States: An Historical Perspective." In R. H. Williams and Lucy D. Ozarin (Eds.) *Community Mental Health: An International Perspective* (San Francisco: Jossey-Bass, 1968).
6. Faris, R. E. and Dunham, H. W., *Mental Disorders in Urban Areas* (Chicago: University of Chicago Press, 1939).

7. Group for the Advancement of Psychiatry, *The Dimensions of Community Psychiatry* (New York: GAP, 1968) Report No. 69, Vol. 6.

8. Kellam, S. G. and Schiff, S. K., "The Woodlawn Mental Health Center: A Community Mental Health Center Model," *Social Service Review*, 1966, 40, 255-263.

9. Keniston, K., "How Community Mental Health Stamped out the Riots (1968078), *Trans-action*, 1968, 5 (July-August), 21-29.

10. Keniston, K., "We Have Much to Learn from Youth," *American Journal of Psychiatry*, 1970, 126, 1767-1768.

11. Kennedy, J. F., *Message from the President of the United States Relative to Mental Illness and Mental Retardation*, House Document No. 58, 88th Congress, 1st Session. (Washington: GPO, 1965).

12. Klee, G. D. *et al.*, "An Ecological Analysis of Diagnosed Mental Illness in Baltimore," in R. R. Monroe, G. D. Klee, and E. B. Brody (Eds.) *Psychiatric Epidemiology and Mental Health Planning*, Psychiatric Research Report No. 22, American Psychiatric Association (New York: APA, 1967).

13. Knowles, M. S., "Some Key Theoretical Issues in Inservice Training," Regional Conference for Planning Inservice Training Programs for Mental Health. 1963, mimeo.

14. Langer, T. S. and Michael, S. T., *Life Stress and Mental Health*. (New York: Macmillan Co., 1963).

15. Leighton, Dorothea C., Harding, J. S., Macklin, D. B., Macmillan, A. M., and Leighton, A. H., *The Character of Danger*. (New York: Basic Books, 1963).

16. NIMH, *Status Report—Community Mental Health Centers Staffing Grants*, NIMH, 1968, p. 11.

17. Pasamanick, B., Roberts, D. W., Lemkau, P. W., and Kreuger, D. B., "A Survey of Mental Disease in an Urban Population—I," Prevalence by age, sex and severity of impairment. *American Journal of Public Health*, 1957, 47, 923-929.

18. Rogers, E. S., "Man, Ecology, and the Control of Disease," *Public Health Reports*, 1962, 77, 755-762.

19. Ryan, W., "Preventive Services in the Social Context: Power, Pathology, and Prevention," In B. L. Bloom and D. P. Buck (Eds.) *Preventive Services in Mental Health Programs* (Boulder: Western Interstate Commission for Higher Education, 1967).

20. Smith, M. B., "The Revolution in Mental Health Care—A Bold New Approach?" *Trans-action*, 1968, 5 (April), 19-23.

21. Yolles, S. F., "Past, Present and 1980: Trend Projections," In L. Bellak and H. H. Barten (Eds.) *Progress in Community Mental Health* (New York: Grune and Stratton, 1969) Vol. 1.

2: Professional and Subprofessional Training in Community Mental Health as an Aspect of Community Psychology

Ira Iscoe

Introduction

Before discussing the topic of training, an attempted clarification of terminology may be helpful. There are currently many intra and interdisciplinary terms related to the field of mental health. Community psychiatry and social psychiatry, community mental health and community psychology are bandied about almost interchangeably. This is understandable in a relatively new, rapidly developing area in which various disciplines are attempting to stake out a claim, each openly declaring the need for interdisciplinary cooperation, yet each understandably striving for its own autonomy. From a strategic sense it would seem that each of the mental health professions is in some way trying to preserve "the best of the old" intermixed with the flood of new behavioral science knowledge that is being generated.

For the purposes of this paper community psychology is viewed as a broadbased endeavor rooted in bahavior science, addressing itself to the analysis of social systems, interventions and social planning. There is a "step back" philosophy, that is to say, community psychology is less concerned with the rendering of mental health services and more concerned with dealing with causal factors. It stresses effective coping by target populations. It definitely hopes for the involvement of the consumer of psychological services, and it has with it a futuristic orientation. Community mental health is subsumed under community psychology and in its broader aspects is concerned with positive mental health, and in its narrower aspects concerned with the delivery of mental health services to persons demonstrating various types of psychological difficulties. Clinical psychology is a narrow spectrum of activities designed to deal with psychopathology of individuals and groups in terms of various treatment and diagnostic procedures.

In all of this it should be remembered that psychology as a profession, as opposed to an academic discipline, is barely twenty years old. Psychotherapy, the chief weapon in the armamentarium of the clinical psychologist, has been questioned as to efficacy. In the area of the poor and in the general malaise of the urban condition, community mental health and community psychology confront their greatest challenges.

Background of Community Psychology

Although the term mental health has been with us for a fairly long period of time, it has only recently taken on more positive connotations. In this respect the mental health professions must acknowledge their indebtedness to the work of Lindemann (1944, 1956) and to the later work of Caplan (1959, 1961, 1964). Their emphasis on the concept of crisis and of the consultant relationships was a great step forward and recognized the potential efficacy of caregivers in the mental health scheme of things.

The Mental Health Studies Act of 1955 established a Joint Commission on Mental Health and Mental Illness. Psychologists were involved in many of the studies carried out under the auspices of the Commission. The Mental Health Manpower Study by Albee (1959) made predictions with regard to shortages in all the mental health fields. These predictions have been borne out in the last ten years. His subsequent call for new approaches to manpower utilization and for new strategies of training are only now beginning to have their full impact. It is of interest to note the precursors of community psychology and a changed strategy in the following quote from Albee:

What we need are techniques and methods enabling far more people to be reached per professional person. If we do not at present have such techniques then we should spend time looking for them. The logic of the manpower situation in which we find ourselves makes other solutions unrealistic.

Any efficient utilization of mental health personnel probably is going to involve something other than time-consuming, face-to-face relationships between a single professional person and a single patient. The number of people who need help and the number of people prepared to give help are so out of proportion that time and arithmetic will not permit such individual face-to-face approaches to be meaningful from a logistics point of view. Perhaps experience in the epidemiology of other disorders will suggest solutions. Just as typhoid fever was never brought under control by treating individual cases of the disease, but rather by discovering and taking steps to remove the source of the disease, so we may find that time might be spent more effectively in prevention, in research, or in public health approaches to mental disorder.[2,3,4]

The publication of the Final Report of the Joint Commission on Mental Health and Mental Illness made a series of recommendations of extreme importance to community mental health and community psychology. Included were the recommendations that mental health facilities be established in community settings, that the manpower base of psychotherapy be broadened, that consultative services be developed and utilized, and that preventive services be instituted. The passage of the Mental Health Facilities Act of 1963 providing funds for construction of facilities as well as supportive staff led to the present growth of community mental health centers throughout the United States. The position paper of the American Psychological Association cautioned against some of the developing trends in community mental health centers. The paper specifically warned against the extension of established notions of clinical psychology and treatment. The community orientation of the paper is unmistakable. The offering of "psychiatry to the community" without a drastic reconceptualization was warned against. The emphasis on more efforts with children and their families was stressed. In retrospect it comes somewhat as a jolt to realize the present great shortages in child clinical psychology. It comes as even more of a shock to realize that present clinical psychology training programs for the most part do not even require Child Development as part of their training or theoretical backgrounds.

The Emergence of Community Psychology

The Swampscott (Boston) Conference of 1965 is appropriately viewed as the place where community psychology was coined. It was at this meeting attended by top-level successful clinical psychologists that broader conception of mental illness and expanded roles for psychologists were envisioned. The Boston Conference may be viewed as a significant point for proposed role changes for clinical psychologists. It expressed dissatisfaction with present approaches and began to deal with possible changes in the academic and field training preparation of psychologists. It recognized that the community was for the most part unknown territory for psychologists. They were comfortable in their clinics and their hospitals. They made occasional forays into mental health associations, but generally they were pretty naive about the organizational processes of communities or for that matter "how things got done" in communities. Since the Swampscott Conference there has been an upsurge of interest in the community, such interest increasing every year.

Clinical psychology arose at the end of World War II in response to the need to treat psychiatric casualties in the military. Veterans Administration training programs and later on NIMH supported programs furnished the bases upon which eventually some seventy APA approved clinical psychology training programs were based. The scientist professional model originally propounded in the Boulder Conference and later reaffirmed has generally guided the training. It should be pointed out that the clinical psychologist was prepared for circumscribed tasks. There was generally the implication of a "triple threat," namely, diagnostic testing, psychotherapy, and research. That the great majority of clinical psychologists have prospered is easily evidenced. That there should be some dissatisfaction with these roles and with prosperity is perhaps a commentary on the effects of behavioral science training and the humanistic bent of some psychologists. The expanded conceptions of mental health and the expansion of support for mental health activities make it impossible to continue in the old vein. The illness model upon which most of the clinical psychology training after World War II was based has not proved conceptually adequate for the task of positive mental health. There have been many attacks upon this model, most notably those of Albee (1967). The disease model demands a tremendous amount of trained manpower, manpower that cannot easily be trained and whose efficacy in a disease model of mental illness is increasingly open to question. Indeed it would seem that the whole question of mental illness is becoming less important and that the establishment of community mental health centers has resulted in the understandable difficulty of distinguishing between *psychopathology* and *social pathology*. Roen (1967) has observed that the basic focus of psychology has changed from what is the nature of man to what are the problems of man. Problems of living exist not only in the psyche of human beings but also in their everyday worlds. The role of environmental factors, especially amongst the poor, is receiving more emphasis.

Community mental health centers with their concept of "zones" have automatically tended to bring problems of social pathology into the mental health clinics. In fact, the zone concept has also brought school systems, policemen, religionists, city councils and politicians. In short it has brought the centers of community power into the mental health field. There is some comfort here that if all this is disconcerting to the clinical psychologist trained in individual psychotherapy and diagnostic techniques, it is almost equally shattering to psychiatry and even to social work. Lastly the burgeoning community psychology movement begins to recognize that whereas in the past "demand" was being met, more attention has to be paid to "need." It is almost axiomatic that as one establishes mechanisms need rises and almost becomes demand. In community psychology the prediction of need or the meeting of need by innovative methods is a prime challenge. It also recognizes that there are emergent mental health needs. The somewhat naive hopes about treating children early in life and preventing mental illness has given way to a probablistic model which recognizes that individuals can be helped in terms of their coping with problems and that at certain times in life even well-adjusted, smoothly functioning human beings may be faced with problems beyond their coping skills. The training of manpower then must take into account these orientations.

The Nonprofessional Sector

The needs of human beings and communities will not be held in abeyance until professional inter and intra-jurisdictional disputes are settled. Human beings adapt to problems. Not all of these adaptations are beneficial, but some have been quite ingenious. In some way or another people will cope. The unmet mental health needs of the nation cannot afford to be ignored. To do so is to commit professional suicide in the sense of divorcement from community support and community regard. Painful though it may be, professionals are beginning to recognize that many of their most sacred ministrations with regard to human beings can be carried on by relatively less well-trained or even untrained persons. The urgency is such that professionals can no longer afford to seek sanctuary in terms of jurisdictional privilege. It has been facetiously said that if Alcoholics Anonymous waited for the blessings of various professionals, it would never have gotten started. Although there is much criticism of Alcoholics Anonymous, there does not appear to be any evidence that indicates that it does any less effective job than more traditional approaches. In fact in some ways Alcoholics Anonymous is now traditional and old hat to seasoned professionals. Certainly A.A. dealt and is dealing with a public health problem that has received too little attention by psychologists. There is also emerging some approaches to narcotic and drug dependency. Certainly the abysmal record of traditional approaches prompts at least an objective examination of the results of organizations such as Synanon, Phoenix, and even the Black Muslims. It is within this area of utilization of nontraditional resources that community psychology faces one of its greatest challenges. What roles is it to play? How is it to intervene in social systems? At what levels? How can top level behavioral science research be separated from do-goodism? What is to be the appropriate academic base and training locus?

Some Choices for Psychology

Forays into the messy field of application and community involvement are admittedly painful especially for the inexperienced. In espousing community involvement it is essential for psychologists not to attack their colleagues who "do not wish to get involved." Community mental health is a value judgment. Those who believe in it should pursue it. Learning studies of sophomores, rats, mathematical models and a detached view of the world have their virtues as well as their rewards and certainly have their place within a university setting. Psychology has not had much experience in the training of persons of various professional levels. There have been symposia upon symposia addressed to manpower needs, subprofessional training, variations in the Ph.D. degree, the involvement of indigenous nonprofessionals, the training of mental health technicians, volunteer therapists and the like. A variety of training programs are currently beginning and Golann (1970) reports there are increasing signs that Ph.D. programs are taking on a mental health flavor if not necessarily a community psychology flavor. Psychologists are "getting involved." The crucial question is at what level and how?

Manpower for What?

Confronted with shortage and expanding need, there is an understandable tendency for a sort of reflex action to training "more of the same"; that is, to beef up the number of people getting Ph.D's and M.A.'s. There is also an understandable tendency to train specialists such as testers, behavior modifiers, group therapists, marriage specialists, sensitivity group leaders, mini-lab conductors, and the like. All of these people have a role to perform. However, a clear distinction should be made between service activities, preventive activities and research. It has been said that one of the greatest challenges of the 20th Century will be the development of a technology of mental health that allows for the fullest development of human beings and permits harmonious relationships between groups and nations. This somewhat trite phraseology however is moving closely to a grim reality. In the last few years we have seen the deterioration of the urban condition, riots, drug abuse, the sexual revolution, the generation gap and the like. Certainly trained manpower is needed to help deal with the casualties of social systems but also trained manpower is needed to begin to unravel the complexities of social systems that produce the casualties. A drastic rethinking of roles, goals and strategies is in order. While there can be no real quarrel of training of people at a technical level, there is certainly much quarrel as to where the technician will be trained and what should be his academic background. For example, in the field of behavior modification or in the setting up of a token economy in a state hospital ward personnel have been shown to be quite effective. Is a college education necessary for these people? Does education beyond a certain degree reduce the empathy and communication between ward attendants and their charges? These are questions for research and legitimately so.

There are other issues that will not vanish in the night. Should technicians be trained without some consideration for the technological changes that are bound to arise? For example, behavior modification may very well give way to some new approach. There may be computer directed psychotherapy. Who will assume the responsibility for the technological upgrading of technicians? Likewise there is the whole question of how will these people be classified. Who will control them and what status will they have as subprofessionals? At this point it is instructive to remember that psychology has had very little experience in the training of technicians. The closest it has come is in the production of an M.A. level person specializing in psychometry or doing psychotherapy "under supervision." Given the nature of graduate training programs today and the general deemphasis of M.A. level training, it seems most unlikely that prestigous universities will become involved in the manpower issues at less than Ph.D. level. It seems most likely, therefore, that less prestigous universities and state and junior colleges will be the key sources of training. Who is to train these people at present remains very unclear. Much depends upon how serious psychologists are about the community. Another aspect that will have to be considered is the use of the term psychologist. It may very well be that this term will be used quite restrictively basing permission for its usage on at least an M.A. degree. If so then the manpower for community psychology will be selected and shaped to meet these needs.

Some Future Perspectives

There is much danger in prematurely crystallizing manpower goals and roles. In a period of ferment and change it would be well not to commit resources to rigid programs and get trapped as the clinical psychologists were twenty years ago. If the goals are merely to produce more manpower to render better care and service to the mentally ill, then the task is relatively simple. Train more aides, use more volunteers, expand consultation services, set up token economies, establish therapeutic communities, work closer with other disciplines. All this is being done to some degree and more or less successfully. In such complex ventures it is doubtful whether we can really know for certain what combination of professional, subprofessional and nonprofessional resources were most effective in achieving improvement in the target populations. It is doubtful whether one can claim that college students as volunteers really made a difference in the status of chronic mental patients without also taking into consideration the attendant changes in the attitude of the hospital, the relatives, and the increased regard by other professionals of the patients. This is obviously a researchable area as are many others in community psychology.

Turning from the subprofessional to the Ph.D. level community psychologist, there is need to acknowledge the unchartered waters that have to be navigated. Will the great bulk of the community psychologists of the future come from modified clinical psychology programs? At this present writing most every mental health facility welcomes a psychologist with community mental health experience. This experience is pretty much ill-defined and so great is the need that minimal experience with a school system, a community action program, a recreational program and the like are acceptable. There are no advertised positions for community psychologists known to the writer.

The role of a change agent, of an intervener, and of a social systems analyst is not an easy one and established community resources do not welcome radical innovations. How to constructively intervene and how to take a long view of a problem are techniques that are just beginning to be taught in some graduate training programs. For the most part community psychology programs are still safely subsumed under community mental health training, or if called community psychology they are community mental health oriented. Although some may decry the present situation it should be remembered that psychologists are relative strangers to communities. Even social psychologists have done relatively little applied work in communities. It is obvious therefore that the background training of Ph.D. psychologists will have to take on more behavioral science and less traditional psychology underpinnings. There are bound to be some painful upheavals within psychology departments, especially established ones. There is the positive impetus of communities impinging upon activities whether universities like it or not. There is also the potential lure of federal and in some cases local funds. There is the deterrent that community mental health centers and communites generally feel that "service" comes first. What kind of psychologist is it, for example, that you pay good money for who doesn't see people? The consultant role is only now becoming halfway accepted and not without its difficulties. The role of the conceptualizer and the planner is more difficult.

There is a well accepted public health maxim that no disease was ever prevented by treating individuals who already had the disease. It would seem that a viable community psychology training program would emphasize preventive and interventive steps. This emphasis on primary prevention will lead higher level trained psychologists into new fields. As Reiff (1970) has pointed out, it may very well be that a new body of knowledge for psychology will have to be generated. It may very well be that current training programs will be drastically modified. It is sometimes forgotten that the Swampscott Conference was only a few years ago. Many things have happened since the Conference, and new developments take place daily. The purpose of this paper has been to point out some of the problems and issues. It offers little or no solutions to the pressing problems of manpower development and training in the mental health and community psychology fields. In some ways many of these problems will be settled not by symposia, but in the market place of human needs. Various training models are urged at various levels, bearing in mind at all times the shortening period between novelty and obsolescence and making provisions for the incorporation of valid research findings. There was never a greater need for hard-nosed evaluation and examination. It is hoped that the appropriately trained manpower will be available for this task. Psychology has gained respect in that it has appropriately been self-critical and willing to examine its theories, its concepts and its procedures. Community psychology must proceed in the same vein. It cannot decry stringent examination and evaluation with the excuse that it is involved with human beings. The public dollar demands accountability in terms of effectiveness. This holds for every level of mental health manpower presently functioning and yet to be developed.

REFERENCES

1. Albee, G. W., *Mental Health Manpower Trends,* (New York: Basic Books, 1959).
2. Albee, G. W., "American Psychology in the Sixties," *American Psychology,* 1963, 18, 90-95.
3. Albee, G. W., "Manpower Needs for Mental Health and the Role of Psychology," *Canad. Psychol.* 1965, 6a, 82-92.
4. Albee, G. W., "The Relation of Conceptual Models to Manpower Needs," In Cowen, Gardner and Zax (Eds.), *Emergent Approaches to Mental Health Problems,* (New York: Appleton-Century-Crofts, 1967) 63-72.
5. Caplan, G., *Concepts of Mental Health and Consultation,* (Washington, D. C.: U.S. Dept. of H.E.W., Children's Bureau Public. No. 373, 1959). (a)
6. Caplan, G., "An Approach to the Education of Community Mental Health Specialists," *Ment. Hygiene,* 1959, 43, 268-280. (b)
7. Caplan, G., *An Approach to Community Mental Health,* (New York: Grune & Stratton, 1961).
8. Caplan, G., *Principles of Preventive Psychiatry,* (New York: Basic Books, 1964).
9. Ewalt, J., *Action for Mental Health,* (New York: Basic Books, 1961).
10. Golann, S. E., "Community Psychology and Mental Health: An Analysis of Strategies and A Survey of Training," In I. Iscoe and C. D. Spielberger

(Eds.) *Community Psychology: Perspectives in Training and Research*, (New York: Appleton-Century-Crofts, 1970).

11. Lindemann, E., "Syptomatology and Management of Acute Grief," *American Journal of Psychiatry*, 1944, 101, 141-148.

12. Lindemann, E., "The Meaning of Crisis in Individual and Family Living," *Teachers College Record*, 1956, 57, 310-315.

13. Raimy, V. C., (ed.), *Training in Clinical Psychology*, (New York: Prentice-Hall, 1950), (The Boulder Conference Report).

14. Reiff, R., "Community Psychology, Community Mental Health and Social Needs: The Need for a Body of Knowledge in Community Psychology," In I. Iscoe and C. D. Spielberger (eds.), *Community Psychology: Perspectives in Training and Research*, (New York: Appleton-Century-Crofts, 1970).

15. Roen, S. R., "Primary Prevention in the Classroom Through a Teaching Program in the Behavioral Sciences." In Cowen, Gardner and Zax (Eds.), *Emergent Approaches To Mental Health Problems*, (New York: Appleton-Century-Crofts, 1967) 252-268.

16. Smith, M. B. & Hobbs, N., "The Community and the Community Mental Health Center," *American Psychologist*, 1966, 21, 499-509.

3: Community Psychology and Public Policy

Robert Reiff

"... the more perfect psychology I dream of will be the acme of humanism. Every human institution will be evaluated by the sole criterion of how much it advances the kingdom of man. On this scale of worths education, art, literature, language, industry, trade, statecraft, law, curative and preventive medicine, philosophy—in short every human institution and invention of man and even the special sciences themselves will be weighed, for the only true and ultimate values in the world are psychological values." [4]

The presence of war, civil disorder and racial conflict, and the failure of some of our fundamental institutions responsible for the socialization of youth are a reproach to psychology and the other social sciences. The failure of organized psychology to respond to these social problems signifies its alienation from people and the social processes by which they live out their lives. But social problems are human problems and nothing human should be alien to the interests and activities of psychologists.

Today our social system is in a severe social crisis. There is every indication that basic changes in social structure and human institutions will result from this crisis. Whether these changes will signal an advance in human welfare or a regression is yet to be decided. It is uncertain whether psychology can have any influence on the course of these changes in the direction of promoting human welfare, but it has the responsibility to make a deep commitment to try. There are a number of groups within psychology who are making such a commitment. But there are also a large number of psychologists who deny the necessity or even the appropriateness of such a commitment. They hold that it is not a "legitimate" activity of organized psychology to influence public policy and programs aimed at solving these social problems. While they are willing to concede that individual psychologists can and should follow the dictates of their social conscience, they act as if psychology as a whole, organized psychology, has only a scientific conscience, as if they were not aware that the Atomic Bomb put an end to the myth of a scientific discipline being responsible only to its science.

For the past several years there has been an increasing demand on social scientists for participation in the solution of social problems. This demand comes from many sources. Community groups struggling for citizen determination and control of human service programs, as well as legislators, public agencies, private and social agencies, program planners in the city, state and federal governments, are all seeking the assistance of social scientists. Social science participation can assume a number of roles—among them, the role of social engineer, that of public educator, or the role of advocate for social forces in the community. The response of psychologists to this demand varies from excitement and enthusiasm at the challenge, through varying degrees of ambivalence, doubt, and reluctance, to open opposition. To many, the invitation is attractive but the responsibility is frightening. Others, feeling they lack the training, experience, and body of knowledge on which to base such activities, would disenfranchise themselves from playing a role in influencing the course and outcome of programs for human betterment in our society, claiming that public policy is an arena for the citizen but not for the scientist or professional.*

Some psychologists who are sympathetic to the purposes and goals of movements for social reform feel that their commitment and participation can be carried out only in their role as citizens. Their psychological knowledge and activity is considered irrelevant or unsuitable. Accordingly, they disenfranchise their scientific or professional selves. Their participation in social change becomes a purely personal concern. Others find a compromise. They, too, hold that

*Throughout this paper the term "public policy" is used in the sense of designating the outcome of the entire political process in the country, not merely in the sense of referring to policies adapted by government at different levels.

public policy choices—the goals and objectives of programs, the setting of priorities and so on—can only be made as citizens, that they are essentially a matter of "political taste." But once the choice has been made, they feel it is justifiable to lend their scientific or professional expertise toward achieving what they desire as citizens.

The question that is being posed is: Should organized psychology, *i.e.*, the scientific and professional components of the discipline of psychology as represented by the American Psychological Association, address itself to the problems of the present social crises? Should it mobilize participation and research for the purpose of contributing to or influencing public policy aimed at solving or alleviating these problems? Put simply, the question is: Does psychology as an organized science and profession have a social responsibility to address itself to social crisis, and if so, what should psychology do?

Professionals as applied scientists think of themselves and their profession as being responsive to, but relatively free of, the influence of social forces. They believe that the manner in which they respond to social forces, the practices they institute to answer a social need, are based on objective, scientific knowledge. They are uncomfortable at the thought that social forces of which they are unaware may not only present the problem to which they respond, but also in part, determine the substantive nature of their response. Thus, the professionals who diagnosed the psychosis of immigrants in the 1850's as "foreign insane pauperism" were convinced they were responding to a contemporary social problem with scientific objectivity. They would be appalled to think that the nature of their response was a consequence of the social and cultural prejudices of their time.

If, in fact, social conditions in part determine the nature of our theory and practice, would we not develop a more objective psychology by becoming aware of the social and cultural determinants of our theory and practice? To make this possible, psychology itself must become the subject of rigorous social analysis.

We will try to demonstrate how this might be done by an analysis of the past activity of organized psychology during periods of social crisis. Our point of view is that social conditions not only influence the activities but the theories of psychology as well. It would certainly be helpful to know, for example, if a relationship exists between certain social and historical conditions and the rise and fall of psychoanalytic theory as the dominant ideology in clinical psychology. Is there a relationship between certain social conditions and the emergence of learning theory or gestalt theory? Such a task, however, is beyond the scope of this book. We are limiting our present analysis to the relationship between social conditions and the *activity* of organized psychology. Assuming that the journals of the past reflect the interests and the activities of the A.P.A. and its membership, we have reviewed those published in times of previous social crises.* The results have yielded some fascinating data which illuminate our present situation and provide a perspective to this problem, free of the distortions which the heat of present social issues invariably introduce.

Organized Psychology and Social Crises

Buckminster Fuller (1963) maintains that all the great advances in human knowledge have come as a result of war. The history of psychology during the last fifty years seems to support this hypothesis. The growth and development of psychology as a profession, *i.e.* an applied science, has been directly related to its activities in the two major wars.

Prior to World War I, psychology was busy consolidating its emergence as an independent discipline from its two historical roots, physiology and philosophy. A review of the early journals, *i.e.*, the *Psychological Review*, first published in 1893, the *American Journal of Psychology*, instituted in 1887, and the *Psychological Bulletin*, originating in 1904, indicates that in this period psychologists were concerned primarily with defining the parameters of the field and with the study of sensation and perception.

Early issues of the *Psychological Review* contain articles dealing with consciousness, sensation, and animal psychology and much material on neurological and philosophical subjects. As late as 1904, papers read at meetings at the American Philosophical Association were included.

*We are indebted to Mrs. Linda Lyons for her diligent survey and classification of the many papers in the Journals of the A.P.A.

The experimental focus of the *American Journal* of *Psychology* is indicated by the predominance of pieces by Titchener. The format of the *Psychological Bulletin* in the first years of publication consisted of several long papers, usually on sensation and perception, reviews of psychological and philosophical literature, and summaries of the papers read at the annual meetings of the A.P.A. In an article in the 1905 issue entitled, "Psychological Progress in 1904" (Buchner, 1905), the necessity of expanding the field of psychology was noted. The relevance of work in the areas of cognition, physiology, testing, abnormal and social psychology was discussed.

The First World War (1913-1919)

In 1917, Yerkes (1917) boldly proclaimed, "among the many scientific problems which the war has forced upon the attention of our military authorities, there are several which are either psychological or present a psychological aspect. In the opinion of experts, many of these problems are immediately soluble and it therefore becomes the *duty* (our emphasis) of professional psychologists to render national service by working on such problems. For this reason a committee on psychology has been organized with the approval of the council of A.P.A. . . . it is the function of this general committee to organize and in a general way supervise psychological research and service in the present emergency." Yerkes urged that psychologists volunteer to serve on whatever committees seemed relevant to their field of interest. Committees were formed to deal with psychological literature related to war, examination of recruits, selection of specific tasks, problems of incapacity, aviation, recreation, discipline, emotional instability, acoustics and vision.

The survey of the literature during this period indicates a substantial shift in focus. The decline of interest in Titchenerian theory, the rise of Behaviorism, refinements of testing procedures, and most important, the focus upon the war, brought substantial changes in the field of psychology. During this period experimental work expanded to include much research in the area of testing. Articles dealing with philosophy began to disappear from the journals. Those dealing with applied psychology substantially increased. Of the 41 papers presented at the A.P.A. meeting in 1912, eight dealt with comparative psychology, ten with experimental, and fifteen with applied. This interest in educational and testing methods was apparent throughout the period as evidenced by the number of papers on these topics presented at A.P.A. meetings and published in the journals. Indeed, at the A.P.A. meeting held in 1916, 22 of the 70 papers presented dealt with mental testing. Interest in animal psychology greatly decreased during this period but was to resume after the War. Much of the literature published in the *Psychological Bulletin* in 1916 pertained to some aspect of the War.

The 1918 publication of the *Psychological Bulletin* discussed methods of army personnel classification, the importance of understanding man in a group, and the learning process, motivation, and leadership problems associated with the war effort. All but one of the papers presented at the A.P.A. meeting in 1919 dealt with problems relating to the war effort.

By 1918 the major interest and activity of psychology was in applied psychology. In 1919, Hall stated that "applied versus pure psychology has abundantly justified itself in this war." Problems related to rehabilitation of the disabled paved the way for the development of rehabilitation psychology, and testing emerged as a major field of psychology. The adaptation of psychological methods to meet military needs was regarded as the primary social responsibility of organized psychology.

The Period of the Great Depression and Recovery (1929–1940)

Between 1929 and 1937, *Psychological Abstracts* lists 10 studies on prohibition and 39 studies on unemployment, in contrast to 83 child development studies, 174 animal studies, and a total of 665 papers on learning!

During this period, renewed interest in animal psychology became evident. Psychology's interest and activity in the areas of testing and developmental and educational psychology broadened considerably.

At the 1930 meeting of the A.P.A., behavior problems of children were discussed and at this point we begin to see interest in the establishment of laboratories for child study. Research dealing with testing methods was widespread. Because of the many refinements of procedures and techniques which had been made, testing methods were applied and extended to the fields of personality, child development, industry, etc. Thurston, in his address to the A.P.A. in 1933, discussed the usefulness of factor analysis applied to vocational aid, attitude study, and psychiatric evaluation. The literature of this period broadened considerably to include material dealing with crime, mental health, and industrial psychology. Five years after the onset of the depression, the A.P.A. Presidential Address in 1935 dealt with psychology as an applied science and the necessity of contributions to government and public questions. At about this time, also, a committee on psychology of the National Advisory Council on Radio and Education was formed, indicating an interest in reaching the general public on a broader scale.

There was at the beginning of this period some interest in social psychology. But few articles were presented dealing with this area, and the role of social psychology was still being defined as late as 1936, when a discussion took place at the A.P.A. attempting to delineate the substantive concerns of social psychology.

The *Journal of Abnormal and Social Psychology* from 1937 to 1940 contains few, if any, articles dealing with the relevance of psychology to social issues. In general, during the whole New Deal period in which many institutions and innovations in government policy were initiated, there is little in the literature relevant to these social changes and reforms.

World War II

In 1940 with the formation of the Advisory Committee on Personnel Problems of the National Research Council, the first formal step was taken to mobilize psychological resources behind the war effort. In that year, the Emergency Committee in Psychology of the National

Research Council was instituted to study sensory problems. Beginning in 1941, psychologists worked on pilot, bombardier, and navigator selection, on problems of sonar operators, fire control, acoustics and optics, and on morale.

Cartwright's review of the World War II activities of psychologists (1947) notes the growth of social psychology during this period. He observes that just as the First World War witnessed the establishment of psychological testing as a major field of psychology, the Second World War brought to maturity social psychology. "Perhaps the most salient feature of the trend of social psychology since 1939 has been an increasing involvement of social psychologists as psychologists in the social problems of the day . . . by and large, the increasing involvement of psychologists in practical problems of social technology was a necessary part of the war."[2] He also points out that during the war most social psychologists were active in government services and served frequently as consultants on specific projects. Stemming in part from refinements in research methods during the late 1930's, the demand grew for social psychologists and many entered the field from other areas of specialization. There was a high degree of interdisciplinary cooperation during the war with a substantial number of projects carried out through the joint efforts of social psychologists, sociologists, and anthropologists. From 1942 until 1945, most of the research was directly related to the war. The 1942 yearbook of SPSSI was devoted to problems of morale and how to combat demoralization. Psychologists conducted many studies dealing with minority group problems within the ranks and the effect of rumor within the civilian population. Psychological warfare was an important activity.

Propaganda policy was determined by pscyhologists. They monitored foreign broadcasts and designed training programs in the field of international relations. They conducted surveys of public needs and popular attitudes and studied and recommended programs to cope with the psychological problems of wartime economy. Following Lewin's theories of democratic organization, a number of psychologists addressed their research to the training of democratic leaders. There were studies to remedy deficiencies in production and to increase worker productivity. Research to prevent and control rumors was also conducted. Public opinion polls were conducted by psychologists to provide civilian intelligence to government and military officials.

In the latter war years and in the early post-war period, clinical psychology experienced a tremendous growth. Clinical psychologists were used to solve army personnel problems and to provide the army with personality information about the individual soldier. Some clinical psychologists were utilized in psychiatric and rehabilitation work. In the immediate post-war period, the employment of clinical psychologists in the Veterans Administration hospitals gave another lift to clinical psychology. It was, of course, during this period that clinical psychology really came into its own, and the need for clinical psychologists in V.A. hospitals led to government sponsored training programs.

Thus we see that the Second World War resulted in a great expansion of psychology especially in the areas of experimental, social and clinical psychology. Again as in World War I, however, this expansion was the result of the application of psychological knowledge and techniques to problems relating to the success of the war effort.

It goes without saying that in the periods reviewed, as in every social crisis, there were individuals and even groups of psychologists who did not share these professional interests and activities or who even opposed them. But the major thrust of psychology as an organized profession is evident and can be succinctly summarized.

The First World War gave birth to psychology as an applied science. There was a rapid adaptation of psychological methods and knowledge to the military needs of the country. This led to the emergence of new roles for psychologists, primarly those having to do with the measurement of capacities and assessment of individual differences in capacity.

The Second World War legitimated psychology as an applied science, gave it official recognition, and established it as a profession as well as an academic discipline. This was symbolized in 1944 by an official act of the American Psychological Association amending its constitution to redefine the objective of the Association. The original objective had been the "advancement of psychology as a science." This was now broadened to encompass two other goals and to read: "The objective of the A.P.A. shall be to advance psychology as a science, as a profession, and *as a means of promoting human welfare* (our emphasis)."[6]

Organized psychology's response to the social problems created by the war and massive mobilization of its resources were immediate. Psychology, like all the other professions, placed itself voluntarily at the disposal of the military in the name of social responsibility. All the principled arguments which in the past and still today are advanced for not responding to social problems were forgotten. Few, if any, opposed wartime activities on the grounds that psychologists should be pure scientists, not practitioners. or that psychologists did not have sufficient knowledge on which to base recommendations, or that value judgments would have to be made. Nobody asked "What is psychological?" about such activities as advising the Office of Civilian Requirements of the War Production Board that the shortage of bobby-pins was quite bothersome to women and that it could be relieved by using less strategic material (Cartwright, 1947). Nobody doubted the value of action research in natural settings. In fact, it suddenly became the most desirable and feasible kind of research. The difficulties of cooperating with other disciplines such as sociology and anthropology which seem to bog us down today became manageable difficulties. Those psychologists who remained in the universities did not criticize their students and colleagues for responding to the social needs created by the war. Organized psychology, *i.e.*, the A.P.A., was not merely responsive to the social need but assumed the initiative in mobilizing psychological personnel and resources.

The legitimacy of influencing government programs and policies was taken for granted by the A.P.A. Psychologists served as consultants and program planners in every branch of government. Some even assumed responsibility for top government and military policies. Psychologists served as advisors to the President of the United States, to military governors in foreign lands, and to such government bodies as the Department of Agriculture, the Morale Services Division of the Foreign Broadcast Intelligence Service, and the Civilian Relations Division of the Office of Civilian Requirements.

Whether one does or does not agree with Buckminster Fuller's thesis, it seems evident that the major wars were the only social crises which sparked a voluntary mobilization of organized psychology.

In contrast to the war years, the interest and activity of psychology during the years of the great depression and recovery period reflect a relative lack of concern with the social problems and needs of that period. During the depression period there was a revival of the pure versus applied psychology controversy. The old "principled" arguments for "scientific objectivity" became popular again. The lack of concern with, even opposition to, applying psychological methods to pressing social problems was widespread. Even those psychologists who were already functioning as applied psychologists continued in the main to utilize their skills in the conventional settings—industry, the academic community, the military or the hospital. Neither the "scientific" nor the "applied" component of psychology lent its talents to studying or working in the natural settings of Hoovervilles, Bread Lines, and public works projects.

To be sure a small group of psychologists did address themselves to pressing social problems. Seven years after the onset of the Depression these psychologists finally realized their organized expression in the Society for the Psychological Study of Social Issues with 333 members.

From these observations of the interest and activity of organized psychology, several patterns emerge which enable us to understand the current controversy within psychology over the question of participation in influencing public policy.

It seems clear, to begin with, that ever since World War I and the birth of applied psychology, organized psychology has contained within itself two functional communities, i.e., the community of scientists-academicians and the community of applied scientists and practitioners. These two communities, unfortunately, developed into conflicting interest groups, but during periods of war their differences were suppressed and an integrated effort made. Between wars the controversy between these two components has persisted over a period of fifty years without any fundamental resolution. In fact, the very same arguments made fifty years ago are still being made today. One reads the eloquent speech of G. Stanley Hall on "Relations between the War and Psychology" delivered at the A.P.A. in 1918 with the feeling that it was written for the A.P.A. meeting in 1968. Anyone of the following statements, for example, could appropriately be written by the next pres dent of the Division of Community Psychology. To the psychologists of today who argue that there is no place in the ghetto for psychology, the voice of Hall from fifty years ago replies, "If there is such a thing as pure psychology, as we speak of pure mathematics, it is an iridescent dream of a goal that is yet very far off, or like the conception of pure soul apart from the body. Its practical domain is daily life. Psychology lives, moves, and has its being in explaining how and why human beings, especially man, sense the world and think, feel, and act in it, and our goal is to control these processes." [4]

To those who question whether psychology should concern itself with social change, Hall answers, ". . . there is a tendency now to reevaluate, analyze, and reeducate the public soul which should be taken full advantage of." [4] On action research, Hall says, "[Psychology's] chief interest is in description and observation, under control of conditions if possible, but it finds precious and still more numerous data where nature and life alone make the conditions, as *e.g.,* in this war." [4]

To those who question whether psychology is a science or a profession, Hall says, "Our science is essentially pragmatic. Its criterion is service. Its supreme end is to teach how to get the most and very best out of life. It may help every science but it can never aspire to be a science apart and by itself, and its history is strewn with the wreckage of futile efforts to attain finalities and hyperexactitude. All such efforts help for a time but in the end retard. They make us feel that we have arrived when in fact we only just started. Ours is the highest, largest, and most complex of all the sciences and will be the very last to approach completeness, which indeed it can never attain until man ceases to develop." [4]

It is indeed surprising to see how eloquently Hall argued 50 years ago against the very same arguments that are being made today by those who resist the demands being made upon psychology to assist in the solution of our society's pressing problems. It is clear, however, that the present controversy has deep historical roots and is part of a pattern. Unless we understand that pattern, there is little chance to break it and move forward. That pattern has the following characteristics:

1. During periods of major war, organized psychology mobilizes itself to respond to pressing social problems created by the war. This thrust results in a rapid growth and expansion of the applied or professional sector of organized psychology. New professional roles and new fields of applied psychology emerge. This does not mean, however, that the scientific sector ceases to exist or become insignificant. Many major theoretical as well as methodological advances were made during World War II, primarily because new forms were created which made possible the integration of the work of scientist and professional among psychologists as well as between disciplines. What was involved was structural change in the institutional settings where psychologists worked. Psychological activity was centered in the locales where the problems existed. Settings were created which were able to harness the energies of both the scientifically oriented and the applied psychologists.

   Since major attention was devoted to the immediate practical solution to problems, the applied or professional sector came to dominate organized psychology.

2. In the post-war periods, there was a return to the old institutional settings. The traditional home of the scientist component of psychology, the university, again became the locale where the bulk of psychological activity was performed. Surely, the new roles and new fields of professional psychology were now larger and more extensive, but they were harnessed to the scientific-academic sector and its institutional settings. Interdisciplinary and intradisciplinary integration of effort broke up. The old controversies and conflicts of interests rose to the surface again. Organized psychology reverted to the old point of view of reluctance, even opposition to responding to social problems.

3. A major war seems to be the *only* social crisis that has led to a mobilization and integration of the scientific and professional components of organized psychology. No matter how severe the social crisis, no matter how pressing the social problems, unless they occurred within the social context of a major war, organized psychology has remained a two-headed creature unable to make an integrated response. Neither Depression, marked institutional

change, racial conflict, or the war against poverty has produced the same response as war. Furthermore, war *itself* as a social problem has never been responded to by organized psychology *during a war*.

Apparently, opposition to participation of organized psychology in the formulation of public policy and programs relating to social problems is not based on any argument of principle. No matter how principled the opponents sound, the history of psychology shows that when major wars occur, organized psychology presents arms.

During World War II considerable work was done for the military on anti-semitism and Negro-white relations for the purposes of morale. Consider, on the other hand, how little has been done on black-white relations during the present crisis. Why is psychology able to advise the government on Negro-white relations to prevent demoralization during the war but seems reluctant or timid, or even opposed to educating the public or advising the government, or assisting black and white organizations to prevent a holocaust in the present social crisis?

The conclusion is inescapable that it is not the social problems per se but the social context in which they occur which determines whether or not organized psychology will respond to them.

Once this is understood, a new problem presents itself. For the question no longer is should organized psychology respond to social problems but rather what are the social conditions, what are the social contexts which determine whether or not organized psychology will respond to social problems.

Why should organized psychology mobilize a massive response to social problems created by a major war and remain indifferent or be opposed to responding to severe social crises at other times? Is it a matter of money? Then how can the fact that psychologists never took advantage of a great deal of money available in the war on poverty be accounted for? Is it a lack of courage? Are psychologists frightened by the violence in the present crisis? But many psychologists heroically risked their lives in war.

The explanation seems to lie in the fact that in a major war every sector of society comes under the domination of the political-military interests of the country. The demand upon psychology is part of a monolithic demand on every available resource in society and all of society is united in its interest in meeting the demand. Under such conditions organized psychology responds with immediate mobilization of its resources, internal tensions and conflicts are suppressed, and a new level of cooperative and integrated activity takes place.

But in times of other kinds of social crisis such as the Depression, the war against poverty, racial conflict, or the failure of our education system, the country is divided. There is no monolithic demand. There are conflicting interests and points of view.

Social problems become social issues and it is impossible to respond to them without taking sides. This is not to say that in the war psychology did not have to take a stand. But taking a stand when everybody is on the same side is vastly different from taking a stand in a divided society marked by controversy and confrontation.

This analysis, then, leads us to the conclusion that there are really no fixed "fundamental" or "principled" objections to psychology's participation in the resolution of social problems. Although the issues are often debated in this way, history shows us that the definition of the "legitimate" role of psychology does not rest on some "ideal" set of values but shifts with the social context in which the issues arise.

When this is a context of controversy, organized psychology retreats to the sidelines. It is a rather interesting morality for a scientific discipline to find it permissible to take a stand on social problems when there is social concensus but to find it not permissible to take a stand on social problems when society is divided. Because the issues in the present social crisis are controversial, the value choices we make, the stand we take, is visible and public.

Now, when called upon to recommend public programs to improve city life, to mitigate racial conflicts, or to eliminate the disabling impact of poverty, psychologists cannot take the position that they can only present the "facts" that have a bearing on these issues but cannot take a stand on specific programs because such a stand would involve taking sides—in other words, making a value choice. Such a separation of "value" and "facts" is no more possible at the present state of the science in areas of public policy than it is in other areas of professional practice. But it is no more "unprofessional" either!

Few today would seriously argue that a value-free science of behavior exists. Built into the very warp and woof of the theories or conceptual frameworks which organize the data in different areas of psychology are implicit value choices.

It is true that the advance of empirical knowledge and the growth of psychology as a science reduce the influence of value judgments on specific decisions. It places constraints in the operation of the value factor and, on a higher level, may at some time in the future make the choice of alternative values, itself, an act resting on scientific knowledge. But today, in the here and now, the overwhelming bulk of our professional practice rests on certain basic value judgments and the great majority of decisions made around specific cases contain not only an empiric but a value component as well.

We can illustrate from many fields that as psychologists, values are involved in our work a great deal of the time. But this is not the image the psychologist presents to the public. He conceals it and negates the value component in decision-making and presents only the empirical-knowledge component. Because he does not make his value judgments visible, the public assumes that his activity consists of scientific judgments only. Once having created this image, we often act as though it were true. Participation in decision-making on social policy does, however, modify one aspect of work. It increases the visibility of the psychologists' value-judgments. But public visibility is not necessarily public accountability. It only makes accountability possible. Responsible professionalism demands making professional judgments visible, explicit, and accountable. Professional practices today often conceal rather than make visible the values which enter into judgments. The present mechanism of professional accountability for professional value judgments is no different than for personal value judgments. It serves to encourage concealment, to create a false image, and promote professional self interest at the expense of public interest.

Psychology cannot shrink from making its value judgments explicit and publicly visible. It is a truism that we are seldom held responsible for mistakes in the dark. We cannot withhold our services because we do not have the protection of the darkness of a private office. Society is asking our help in shaping the course of social programs for human betterment. Psychology must not refrain from participating in public policy and social planning for our society out of fear of exposing its value judgments to public scrutiny or having to be responsible to the public for them. A new mechanism for accountability to the public must be developed. We should welcome rather than fear this development. It does not necessarily entail high risk for organized psychology or lowered status for the individual psychologist.

The fact is that values play a distinctively different role in professional decision-making than they do in nonprofessional decision-making. They are part of an organized conceptual framework and related in some way to empirical data. The professional decision is never "purely" a value decision; it must contain a knowledge component. The nonprofessional judgment can and often is all value—a matter solely of taste or morality whether it pertains to the characterization of an individual (a homosexual has no moral fibre) or a social issue (Legalize Pot!).

If there is no empiric component at all, there is no basis for a professional decision. On a problem or issue where this is the case, a professional has nothing to offer as a professional. It must be acknowledged that there are areas and issues where there is insufficient knowledge to justify professional intervention. Participation as professionals under those circumstances might be irresponsible and misleading, giving rise to the impression that the psychologist's opinion is somehow "better" than someone else's or rests on some foundation other than political preference. We are certainly not in a position to offer our services as consultants to anybody, any place, and on any problem under the sun, to extend the imperialistic flag of psychology over all of society. What is required is to make explicit the basis for our participation in each specific instance.

It would be quite naive to expect that the field of psychology should be the only source of knowledge. Problems that arise in the public arena are never "purely psychological" in nature. Programs involve allocation of funds and thus they have an economic component; organization and implementation of public programs takes place within the political network. Many disciplines and many professional fields may be implicated in, and have a contribution to make to, consideration of a single problem.

The knowledge base for community psychology includes but goes beyond psychology. Neither psychology, nor sociology, nor political science, nor economics can by itself provide a sufficient data base for the solution of most of the pressing social problems of our society. Society is asking psychology to play a role in the process of shaping public policy. It is not asking psychology to take it over.

Many clinicians and other psychologists are bringing to Community Psychology an empirical body of knowledge from their own specialty. The process involves a reorganization of their experience and knowledge of their specialty to new problems, problems of social policy, community planning, and program development to mention a few. This reorganization also involves the integration of empirical knowledge from other professions and from outside the professions altogether, from history and philosophy and from the organizational experience accumulated in practical life activities. The reorganization of these various data bases should ultimately result in a fairly substantial body of knowledge for community psychology.

Another argument raised by those who question psychology's participation in policy-making is that participation in decisions of public policy entail great risk. If the criteria for participating in making decisions is going to be a guarantee that we know beforehand we are right, we will not be able to participate in any decisions whether they be decisions about individuals in therapy or how to promote civilian morale. There is, of course, a hidden preconception here. People often operate on the false assumption that decisions merely involve the making of a choice between right or wrong or a good or bad course of action and that once the decision is made it will turn out to be good or bad, right or wrong, without any further action or intervention on their part. There is a general attitude that making a decision about some course of action or some social problem is similar to calling heads or tails or picking a winning horse. There is a general feeling that once a decision is made, the die is cast. But decisions that have to be made regarding social problems and public policy are not the kind of decisions which simply involve one in casting a die. They are more commonly the kind of decisions in which one really decides to cast his lot with a particular course of action. To cast one's lot means to commit oneself to making every effort to influence the course of events so that the desired result may occur. Decisions on public policy are not fatalistic decisions. They are, in effect, guidelines for action to achieve a desired goal. They involve setting the directions in which energies are to be mobilized to make the decisions come out right.

The truth of the matter is that it is not the risk to the public that psychology is primarily concerned with, but the risk to itself in having to place its judgments on the line, to make its values explicit and visible to the public.

If the social crisis appears to require extensive changes in our institutional structure, there is the risk of incurring the wrath of the establishment in these institutions. This is the real risk; the one that really lies behind the reluctance of organized psychology to commit itself to a program of participation in social change. But at least for the present, there are many forces within the establishment in government and other institutions who realize that basic social change is necessary and who desire the professional help of psychology. The risk of sanctions is not very great today. But, the political situation may change in the future and a great opportunity will have been wasted.

The risk is also a challenge. Can psychology commit itself to becoming an applied science devoted to "promoting human welfare" in a society torn by conflicting interest and survive without compromising itself?

It is doubtful if it can remain unresponsive to social problems. In fact, it has already shown some movement toward addressing itself to some of these problems, usually under pressure from some group within psychology or from public opinion. Basically, it has been only reactively responsive. It has been reluctant to take the initiative and mobilize its resources to respond to the present social crisis. If, in times of national wars, it is legitimate for organized psychology to declare the highest priority to, and to mobilize its resources for, the military, it is certainly legitimate for it in times of national internal crisis to declare the highest priority to, and mobilize its resources for, psychology's contribution to these internal social problems. For example, there are a number of psychologists today who, following the old pattern, are placing their services at the disposal of the military in the present war and internal crisis.

The Department of Defense spent 40 million dollars in the fiscal year

1968 for Behavioral and Social Science research. Should organized psychology ignore this situation, or should it in the interest of human welfare examine the substantive nature of the research and take a position on whether or not it is in the interest of human welfare?

A memorandum from the Board of Scientific Affairs of the A.P.A. suggests that a major contribution of the A.P.A. to the public welfare could be a series of white papers which reflect and present the knowledge of our science pertinent to social issues and public policy matters. This is an important step forward. It is one of the ways in which organized psychology can participate in shaping public policy. But how long will it be before this suggestion is implemented. One can only hope that the A.P.A. will move with more than its usual cumbersome sluggishness and delay to set such a program in motion.

In the same memorandum there are comments about the fact that the A.P.A. and the scientific community in general do not speak in an organized and potent manner to the issues of Federal appropriations of funds for research and development. But the approach to this problem is purely negative, i.e., opposition to a cutback in R & D funds. It is at best ambiguous about what it believes the A.P.A.'s priorities should be with regard to appropriations for research, development and training. It is not sufficient to say we are against cutbacks, or even to say we are for more money for R & D and training without specifying also the substantive nature of the psychological research, development, and training that psychology feels should have highest priority in the present social crisis.

Institutions are by nature resistant to change. Fortunately, the A.P.A. is a viable organization which has built into it mechanisms which make it aware of changing needs, i.e., its divisional structure. The Division of Community Psychology is one of these mechanisms. It has declared its commitment to respond to social problems and to pursue social change when its psychological skills and knowledge can contribute to "promoting human welfare." It is a step ahead of organized psychology. But it has yet to implement its declaration and commitment.

Community psychology can become the mechanism which demonstrates to organized psychology the possibilities inherent in a new coalition between academicians and applied scientists. This is necessary to recruit and train community psychologists. On the one hand, the young students need to integrate life experiences in the community with a conceptual framework. This is the real meaning of the participant-conceptualizer.* On the other hand, the universities need continuous and meaningful contact with life in the community. Only through a coalition between academicians and applied scientists working in the community can this be accomplished. Just as new institutions and new settings were created in wartime which made possible a coalition between the scientist-academician and the professional and produced a new level of integration of effort, community psychology can be instrumental in creating new settings and new institutional forms to make possible a new level of psychological activity addressed to social problems.

Community Psychology is not simply the organizational expression of a desire to respond to pressing social problems. The substantive nature of the response, i.e., the emphasis on changing social systems, on action research, on participation in social planning, is also the result of social forces or pressures directly attributable to the social reform movement sparked by the civil rights struggle and the war against poverty.

The central theme of the social reform movement of the past few years has been to increase citizen participation and control of public programs and policies. To effectively participate and control, the public and the government need more knowledge about how to make human institutions more effective for human development. Psychology has a social responsibility to respond to their needs.

For this reason community psychology is commited to mobilizing psychological resources for the purpose of addressing itself to questions of public policy and participating in shaping it.

REFERENCES

1. Buchner, E. F., "Psychological Progress in 1904," *Psychological Bulletin,* 1905, 2, 89-98.

*The concept of Participant-Conceptualizer was first put forward by Forrest B. Tyler at the Swampscott Conference, May, 1965.

2. Cartwright, D., "Social Psychology in the United States During the Second World War," *Human Relations*, 1947, 1, 333-350.
3. Fuller, B., *Ideas and Integrities, A Spontaneous Autobiographical Disclosure*, Marks, R. W. (Ed.), (Englewood Cliffs, N. J.: Prentice-Hall, 1963)
4. Hall, G. S., "Morale in War and After," *Psychological Bulletin*, 1918, 15, 361-426.
5. Hall, G. S., "Some Relations Between the War and Psychology," *American Journal of Psychology*, 1919, 30, 211-223.
6. Wolfe, D., "The Reorganized APA," *American Psychologist*, 1946, 1, 3-6.
7. Yerkes, R. M., "Psychology and National Service," *Psychological Bulletin*, 1917, 14, 259-263.

4: Health and Disease

Observations on Strategies for Community Psychology

Louis D. Cohen

The crescendo of articles on the medical model and its deficiencies when applied to psychological disorders has reached the point where many psychologists and physicians believe that there is an intrinsic deficiency in the model. It is held that the need now is to identify an entirely new approach to the problem of the psychologically ailing person. What is it about the medical model that generates so much criticism?

At least three aspects of the medical model have been criticized: first, the *nature of the difficulty* challenges the usual and traditional concern of medicine with a biological concept of etiology and pathogenesis; second, *how people are treated* questions the administration and organization of the delivery of health services; and third, *who gives the treatment* is critical of the "medical establishment": the formal and informal social and political structures and relationships which have grown up around treatment, research, and training. Arguments directed against the medical model seem to focus on some admixture of all three of these facets so that it becomes difficult to disentangle the arguments against each.

It may be useful at the outset to illustrate by noting a few positions on this issue. One concept of the medical model is expressed in the statement " ... the individual's behavior is considered peculiar, abnormal or diseased because of some underlying cause," a definition focused on an intrinsic deficit or disorder within the individual. It is rejected as too restricted a statement of illness and limiting of therapeutic intervention.[27]

Another view of the "medical model" asserts that the concept is not appropriate to, nor particularly useful for, the "mental" disorders which are seen as arising largely from problems in adaptation to complex social forces, and not at all involving the biological and related considerations usually associated with disease.

Further, the use of diagnostic labels typical of medical practice, when applied to the mental disorders, has a pejorative impact and not the etiological, therapeutic, and prognostic character of the usual medical diagnoses (Szasz, 1960). These pejorative qualities are seen as influencing negatively both the therapist and the patient.

The first position quoted attributes a deficit orientation to the medical model and excludes recognition of the role of ecological and environmental influences. The second position emphasizes social competence and excludes biology.

Brown and Long (1968) have noted this polarity between biological and social domains, but they maintain that these views need not be mutually exclusive, rather that they can be regarded as complementary aspects of the medical model.

The Nature of the Difficulty

I should like to examine some concepts of the nature of disease to see whether the goal of an integration of the polar positions on biological and social models may be elaborated. And it should be said at the outset that much support for such an integration will be found in the history and conceptualizations of medicine (Sigerist 1945, Stainbrook 1961, Engel 1963, Dubois 1965).

Let me indulge in a bit of historical review which may be overly simple but may set the stage for some later remarks.

The recent history of medicine—the period of the past one hundred years—has produced most of the facts we know about the relationship between biological disturbances and disease. One heavy emphasis has been the germ theory, which has been responsible for remarkably useful inputs to our knowledge of disease.

With the advent of the microscope, the determination of the cellular nature of living matter and the identification of microorganisms, the quest over a long period of time was for identification of the invading microorganisms. Each discovery only reinforced the validity of the concept, so that today many people equate disease with the existence of a "germ" or virus, or some other microscopic or submicroscopic particle.

However, this exciting and productive concept of disease has had to bend and be amplified to accomodate new types of data. The deficiency diseases—particularly the vitamin deficiences—were among the earliest dramatic new data to cause a modification in germ theory. Another class of events found to cause disease was that of accident and trauma. Correlative with the study of trauma were the findings that there were many stresses on organisms, ranging from biological to psychological events, that seemed to result in disease. Genetic variations, as in Huntington's chorea, or congenital deformities in consequence of metabolic disturbances in intrauterine life, were also seen as etiologically related to disease. The list can be amplified, but my point here is that disease is known to be at least more than invading microorganisms.

Further amplifications in the concept of disease have become necessary. It is not only the microorganisms but the state of the host organism at the time of invasion and the host characteristics that determines the effect of the microorganism. The person in splendid good health can often combat the microorganism. Some evidence of past successful combat has been noted in people whose routine x-rays of the chest show signs of the battle with the TB bacillus, but no evidence of organismic breakdown.

Perhaps the area of allergic responses may illustrate this point. It is not only the presence of rose pollen, but the special sensitivity of a specific individual to rose pollen that creates the problem. Hypersensitivity or hyposensitivity, however acquired, becomes a variable in the eventual disease response.

Stress is another experience that is particularly dependent upon personal thresholds for specific traumatic events. The sustained exposure to combat nurtures one individual and overwhelms another.

Ambiguity, or conflict, undermines one and is well tolerated by another.

These observations lead us to note that it is not only the external event, but the host resistance—the biological resources, the experiential matrix, and the learned response modes—that make the external event a special disease precipitating occasion.

Thus there seems to be at least two classes of event: the first, largely *external*, includes microorganisms, deprivation or deficiency (as in diet), stress and/or trauma or accident; and the second, *internal*, such as hereditary coding, sensitivities or insensitivities (due to innoculations and similar experiences) and learned modes of response.

These two classes of events interact at any given time. Evidence and theory over the past 75 years suggest that the organism attempts to maintain a balance, a homeostasis, to work out a resolution between the stressors and the resources available for overcoming them. This process of resolution—this adaptational process—may or may not be wholly successful. If it is wholly successful no evidence of disease may result. If it is wholly unsuccessful, impairment or death may result. If adaptation is only partially successful, there may be chronic mal-adaptation, or chronic disease. *Disease itself is the failure of the organism to adapt to the environmental stresses upon it, whether these stressors are primarily biological, psychological, or social in nature. And the evidence of disease, or failure of adaptation, may be noted in a number of experiental domains, be they biological, psychological, or social.*

Students of the history of medicine and of the broad context of illness seem to come to this adaptational view of health and disease. May, (1958) in reporting on The Ecology of Human Disease, notes, " . . . the word disease becomes synonymous with the word 'maladjust-ment'. It expresses a temporary state of the living cell in conflict with environmental challenges and trying to cope with them and survive."[1][7] Dubois (1965) notes, "Ever since Claude Bernard, disease has been regarded by physicians and pathologists as the outcome of *attempts* at adaptation, without regard to the precise mechanism involved, or to the conditions which elicit the response."[7]

The criteria of successful coping are not absolute. Different cultures and subcultures define the specific behaviors idiosyncratically. One culture tolerates giving away all your possessions; another does not. One culture tolerates high rates of alcoholic consumption; another does not. It follows that what is a disease in one culture may not be so regarded in another. To quote from Bloom:[2]

"The causal connection between iodine deficiency and exophthalmic goitre is crystal clear, yet in many places in southeast Asia, goitre is not only endemic with its resultant sapping of human productivity, intellect, and life expectancy, but also its eradication is struggled against by its very victims because of the belief that, without a goitre of optimal size, a Burmese or Laotian or Cambodian woman is not a desirable marriage prospect. The goitre in many parts of southeast Asia, much as the female breast in the United States, has taken on a secondary significance unrelated to and often more important than its original function."

We now seem to have identified four different aspects of this process of disease: the *external* and *internal* variables, the coping or *adaptive skills*, and the *cultural view of the response*.

The process that I have sketched does not distinguish separate biological, psychological, or social domains. All are interrelated in the experience and response of individuals. In the same sense, it becomes difficult to separate a biological disease from a psychological disease. These are different dimensions of the same problem. Stainbrook (1961) has stated the broad framework of the sociocultural context within which disease must be viewed:

"Since there are concomitant physiological processes associated with every individual behavioral event, and since probably no act of individual behavior is unrelated to the social space in which it is occurring, body and society are in a constant transaction across a total field of reciprocal determination. In many constantly shifting patterns, body and person are the environment of society as society becomes the environment of person and body.

Moreover a comprehensive theory of disease, interrelating body, person, human group, and the physical environment signifies, diagnostically, an insistence upon etiologic patterns or fields even if the major search for structural defect or dysfunction is confined to the body. Hence, every disease in some balance of etiological patterning is a psychosomatic, a psychosocial and a bio-social ill-at-easeness.

All these statements are a theoretical prelude to an insistence that much of what goes on inside bodies is intimately related to what goes on between bodies. The understanding of the structures, functions, and values of social organization is not optional and elective for medicine and the public health, but imperative. The sciences of social man and of individual behavior, the behavioral sciences if you will, are an integral part of basic medical science."[24]

The broad definition of disease—this unified conception of health and disease that I have noted—seems consistent with the evidence, but its very breadth may present problems at the level of implementing service. While the adaptational problems of people involve simultaneously their biological, psychological, and social experiences, services to people who are sick are usually provided by physicians whose major interest and focus are on the biological aspects of disease or maladaptation. The psychological or social aspects of disease often get short shrift.

I have noted that a patient who has had an acute cerebral accident resulting in aphasia and hemiparesis will be told after three or four days that his illness has been stabilized and that the physician has done as much as can be done. In effect, the patient is told to go home and resume his duties. But we all recognize that there are a number of aspects of the disease that have not been attended to. The patient is far from able to return to duty, but the physician is through with his contribution. I would contend that our medical training programs and the dominant culture of medical practice encourage this type of action.

Such a practice is generally not condoned by spokesmen for medicine. As Sigerist (1943) has pointed out, "The goal of medicine is not merely to cure disease; it is rather to keep men adjusted to their environment as useful members of society or to readjust them when illness has taken hold of them. The task is not fulfilled simply by a physical restoration but must be continued until the individual has again found his place in society, his old place if possible, or if necessary a new one. This is why medicine is basically a social science."[22]

If, indeed, there is a broad spectrum to the concept of disease we may ask what type of establishment, or what kinds of professionals are, or may be, set up to deal with the patient's problems. If medicine as it is now practiced focuses on the biological aspects of disease, who, if anyone, is concerned with the psychological and social components of illness?

It may also be relevant to note that many diseases may, by their very nature, emphasize one or another component of the spectrum I have described. Chronic alcoholism, which is now being subsumed under the broad definition of disease, can often present more salient concerns for the psychological and social than with the biological aspects of the maladjustment. And interventions for primary biological disturbance may find their answers in psychological and social actions. Again, let me quote from Bloom:

"Beri-beri, a nutritional disease endemic in the Philippines, can be prevented simply by ceasing to remove the hulls and outer layers of rice before preparing it for eating. Yet an extraordinarily resistant strain of folklore has arisen around this somewhat yellowish outer layer which makes this simple preventive device unpalatable."[1]

A Strategy for Community Psychology

Perhaps then a society that wishes to control disease has a number of points at which it can intervene. If we attend to the *nature of the difficulty*, and if we accept the four components that I have noted as relevant to the disease process, we may want to intervene at any or all the points I have described. We may want to provide some inputs to influence or control (1) the external stressors, (2) the host resistances, (3) the adaptational process, or (4) the cultural definitions of disease.

Let us take a closer look at some strategies that might be used in a community psychology program. The first point is that of influencing or controlling the external stressors. Sigerist (1943) says:

"Steady employment under the best hygienic conditions, the correct balance between work, rest and creation, and wages that permit a decent standard of living—these are basic and significant factors in public health."[22]

Among the major influences on health is the general economic status. Analyses of mortality and morbidity data show higher rates for the lower socioeconomic groups of any society. Poor housing, poor temperature control, unclean water, the absence of bathing facilities, poor diet, high pollution indices for air and water, poor waste disposal, poor health care, poor prenatal care, low educational levels, all contribute both to the external pressures on people and to the reduced internal resistance to the pressures.

I am reminded of a story I heard when I was in England during World War II. It was noted then that despite the paucity of physicians for civilian care, the rates of infant and maternal mortality had been reduced during the war years. This somewhat unexpected turn of events lent itself to an explanation. It seemed that during the war, with government control of food distribution, and rationing of eggs, milk, and butter, highest priority was given to pregnant women and nursing mothers. Regardless of economic status, these women were provided with a balanced diet during their special period of need resulting in a drop in infant and maternal casualties.

Control of the environment for the prevention of disease involves a broad range of activities. The economic status of a community, the ethical values of a society, the conduct of social institutions and the concern for the well being of the society's members, the distribution of food, the educational system and its availability to all members of a society—these and similar problems, issues and activities are germaine to considerations of health and well being. But the solutions to some of these problems are the special concern of selected professionals, while other problems are the concern of all citizens. What special role does the psychologist play in preventing disorders of health and well being? How does his competence as a professional give him special entry in contrast with other professionals? To what extent does his competence as a professional overlap with his concern as a citizen? (A more detailed analysis of these issues may be found in a concurrent paper by Robert Reiff in this volume.)

George Miller (1969), in his presidential address to the American Psychological Association, grappled with some of these problems and in particular with the current posture of psychology in regard to human welfare. It was clear from his analyses that psychology had contributed some new insights to the basic conceptions of man, to the strategies for social innovation, and to the professional base for implementing change, but these developments were still emerging. Despite the deficiencies in knowledge and skill, his optimistic view called for a grappling with social problems by psychologists with the hope that social gains would emerge. Miller suggests a point of departure for action:

" . . . in the beginning we must try to diagnose and solve the problems people think they have, not the problems we experts think they ought to have, and we must learn to understand these problems in the social and institutional contexts that define them. With this approach we might do something practical for nurses, policeman, prison guards, salesman—for people in many walks of life."[18]

But perhaps a more fundamental finding is the emerging view of man that psychological science is making possible. The potential consequences of these insights for changing our social institutions is enormous. Miller contrasts two views of man: one, on which our present social institutions are based and another, the product of psychological science. Excerpts from his paper attributed to an unpublished volume by Varela may be pertinent. The first view:

"All men are created equal. Most behavior is motivated by economic competition, and conflict is inevitable. One truth underlies all controversy, and unreasonableness is best countered by facts and logic. When something goes wrong, someone is to blame, and every effort must be made to establish his guilt so that he can be punished. The guilty person is responsible for his own misbehavior and for his own rehabilitation. His teachers and supervisors are too busy to become experts in social science; their role is to devise solutions and see to it that their students or subordinates do what they are told."

The second view: "There are large individual differences among people, both in ability and personality. Human motivation is complex and no one ever acts as he does for any single reason, but, in general, positive incentives are more effective than threats or punishments. Conflict is no more inevitable than disease and can be resolved or, still better, prevented. Time and resources for resolving social problems are strictly limited. When something goes wrong, how a person perceives the situation is more important to him than the "true facts", and he cannot reason about the situation until his irrational feelings have been toned down. Social problems are solved by correcting causes, not symptoms, and this can be done more effectively in groups than individually. Teachers and supervisors must be experts in social science because they are responsible for the cooperation and individual improvement of their students and subordinates."

For the professional psychologist, these observations direct him to working with the social institutions of our society, to the study of their implicit assumptions about man and the consequences of these assumptions, to the management of these institutions and the ways in which this management is facilitated or impeded. We need to pay close attention to the interpersonal processes that influence the functioning of major institutions of the society since the operation of these institutions may have significant effects on the lives of citizens.

Perhaps for these reasons the community psychologist today spends much of his time consulting with the formal agencies of a community to help clarify both its mission and its functioning.

The second point of intervention would be building up resistance as one way of shaping the internal resources to withstand external adversity. Knowing the potency of microorganisms, it is now possible to build up immunization against a large group of potential dangers. Our children at an early age are protected against diptheria, measles, small pox, and many of the scourges of mankind. We adults find it easy now to protect ourselves against typhoid, typhus, yellow fever and cholera and we are reminded of this every time we take off for a visit to a less well-protected geographic area. The principle of building up internal resources to withstand external assault is well illustrated in our lives.

However, the domain of inner resources is not confined to protection against microorganisms. Let us consider the area of stress. We can recognize that the inner resources of the person give special meaning to the specific stressor. Being able to read and write makes the conditions of urban living less stressful. Being skilled and able to get a job and high wages reduces the tensions around adapting to complex social living. Being able to meet the demands for social functioning reduces the stresses on a man. By building up skills and knowledge, we enable ourselves to prevent the crisis that would overwhelm us if we were less well prepared.

Some of the early intervention programs illustrate this point. The "Head Start" program, a public venture in supplementing life experiences for culturally deprived preschool children, is designed to build in better skills and knowledges in these youngsters. And going back even earlier in the life span, Ira Gordon (1969) has been conducting enrichment programs beginning at age 3 months and continuing for some years. These preventive programs are designed to enhance the capacity of the child to adapt and to withstand the stresses of living.

Skill in coping, the third variable, also seems to offer a place for intervention. These skills are the learned social adaptations that are the consequence of experiences in the home, the school, and in the larger society. How one approaches life's problems is a product of these experiences. Whether to look to yourself for some resolution of a problem or to give up helplessly; whether to run away or to confront; and whether options exist for using different methods at different times are the outcome of previous experience.

These skills can be enhanced and the repetory broadened. Some of my colleagues (Sprigle and Van De Riet, 1968), working with Head Start children, have reported an increase in the variety of problem solving strategies used by children after having had a chance to go through a program designed to enhance self reliance and initiative.

Other programs are being developed that illustrate this principle. Cowen, Gardner, and Zax (1967), for example, have worked with one school in which they identified first graders who were having difficulty in adaptation. Using the resources of the professional services in the schools and the community, they designed an intervention program predicated to enhance the skills of these maladapting youngsters. By careful programming they were able over a year or two to improve the coping mechanisms of these youngsters. The program is now being applied to the entire school system.

This early "case finding" and intervention may have value for the eventual prevention of major maladjustment.

The cultural view of disease, our fourth point for intervention, involves an area with which we are familiar. Currently we are seeing a major change in the approach to at least one social phenomenon: alcoholism. Until recent years it was considered a willful defiance of the moral code and was punished by imprisonment. We know of prison systems in which alcoholic offenders have been confined for up to two years for public drunkenness. Now we are beginning to see changes in our posture toward alcoholism. It is beginning to be identified as a disease and as a concern of the health institutions of our society. Our shifting societal criteria takes a behavior out of the criminal class and puts it into the sick class. And since our society shows special favors to the sick, with it goes a change in approach and expectations.

Our approach to mental illness changed similarly about 200 years ago in Western European society. We had viewed mental illness as immoral but slowly have changed our attitudes and consequent treatment methods.

Our view of drug addiction is currently under controversial debate and whether it will be considered immoral or a disease will depend on many social variables.

This sketch of strategies has focused on behavioral disorders. Consistency, and the evidence, would suggest the relevance of such strategies for biological disorders as well.

Thus, I would assert that this conceptual framework provides a schema for integrating the biological, psychological, and social aspects of disease and for identifying potential avenues for intervention. However, many of our difficulties in providing patient or client care, whether by physicians, psychologists, social workers, or other professionals, come not from the conceptual framework about disease, but from the society's organization of services for patients and in the allocation of responsibility for providing services.

How People are Treated

Let us turn, then, to the second major aspect of the medical model—*how people are treated*—or to the administration of health services. It is becoming increasingly clear that some readjustments must be—and are being—made at a national level. The whole fabric of medical care practice is under close scrutiny and criticism both from within and without. Dr. Rutstein says:

"Our pattern of medical care has been with us for more than half a century, has worked well in its time, and has assumed an air of permanence. The physician has been practicing in relative isolation in his home or in a professional building. The hospital has been going its self-centered way, adding beds or facilities at the behest of its staff or at the urging of a trustee. Local health departments, by imposed tradition, have been kept out of the hospital and have been safely isolated in city hall from becoming involved with medical care. Too many people have been receiving their care in inadequate clinics through the charity of the individual physician or from a welfare doctor. The large teaching hospital affiliated with a medical school has been giving high quality impatient care for diseases of interest to its staff while showing little or no concern for the continuity of medical care for the patient before his admission and after his discharge from the hospital . . . But the old edifice is beginning to crumble. More physicians are now working full time in medical schools, in industry, and in government, and many fewer in private practice. Community demands on the hospitals are beginning to make themselves felt. The artificial line between preventive and curative medicine is being obliterated . . . ."[19]

As we have noted earlier, health is now seen as more than medicine or medical care. It is, in part, a product of the social matrix within which people live, and the delivery of health services depends upon this social setting. Within this context, traditional patterns of health care have changed slowly in the face of demands for meeting the new realities of our society. New approaches are being explored with significant consequences in redefined problems of health and in the identification of wider possibilities of action. This is provocatively illustrated in an article by Schaeffer and Hilleboe. Using a systems analysis approach to community health, they trace some potentials for change in emphasis. Beginning with a public health truism, "Public health is, by nature, a problem of changing social behavior,"[21] they spell out some of the consequences of a new approach based on this postulate. They note that the essence of the problem "would consist of altering conceptions, attitudes, and actions on the part of persons, groups (notably families and other basic social units) and communities." Further, "Activities to modify the conceptions and attitudes that underlie behavior must be pursued in diverse forms and at various levels." And, "Administrative adaptations may be found necessary not only in the ways in which services are provided to families, but in the way health organization functions at the community level."[21]

To carry out these newly defined responsibilities, the health agency will have to call upon experts not now usually found in such agencies: " . . . the social psychologist, political sociologist, systems analyst, and others who have a professional contribution to make in changing social behavior." The health officer would function primarily as a coordinator of a wider spectrum of cooperating specialists. More and different professions would be involved in the health enterprise. There would be many professionals not now seen in the "health team", and the internal structure of their relationships would be changing.

The basic change would be in the conception of community health, which would call for a reduction in the boundaries between the official health organization and other community health and welfare agencies. "While the needs of persons and families for education, employment, housing, social status, healthful environment, medical care, and constructive use of leisure time can be intellectually factored and functionally divided for purposes of administrative organization, the problems themselves are unified in persons and social groups."[21]

The theme of the current revolution in health care is the shift in focus from the health of the individual to the health of the community and its members. Such a shift calls for an expansion in the resources for health care and in the variety of professions, skills, and workers involved in the health enterprise. It calls as well for a reorganization of the internal structure of society's agencies and in their interrelationships when directed to the community's health problems.

Fundamental shifts in attitude have precipitated this demand for change. The willingness to think of health services as a right of the citizen and to expect quality care for each citizen presses on a system functioning on an older entrepreneur model.

Psychologists have a responsibility to help in this reorganization—both as citizens and as professionals. As professionals, they will have to tackle some knotty problems. Let me note a few.

Fuchs (1968) sees the most significant need in the health field to be in what people do, and do not do, to and for themselves. And he quotes Colman (1967) in pointing out, "Positive health is not something that one human can hand to or require of another. Positive health can be achieved only through intelligent effort on the part of each individual."[5] How to get each person involved in his own self determination with regard to his health activities can challenge psychologists for some time.

And as Hughes (1966) sees it, the main tasks of medical institutions are "those of maintaining and enlarging the capacity for *living*, living in all its dimensions, those of psychological exhilaration and meaningful social purpose as well as those of sheer bodily virtuosity." He asks, " . . . what good will it do to expand enormously the length of life . . . if this will only mean that large numbers of people can simply be bored with life for that much longer, or that others will suffer the sentiments of alienation and humiliation for more than the 'three score and ten'?"[14] This, too, is a noteworthy challenge to psychology and to the value oriented members of our society.

But, more specifically, we psychologists have been considering for some years the establishment of services for people whose presenting concerns are largely psychological. Among the solutions offered is the establishment of centers for dealing with problems of living. These centers, some few prototypes of which now exist, serve as independent agencies or as parts of community mental health services.

The hope of the problem-of-living center is to deal with problems that are now being confronted with the full resources of professional imagination and skill. If my observations are correct, the present practice of health care leaves these problems of living relatively untouched by medical personnel and social agencies. Indeed, there are many social agencies that get into "the action" — the church, the schools, the courts, the social service agencies—but alleviation of problems of living are usually secondary to the functions of these institutions. In setting up such centers, psychologists see themselves as meeting a serious social need.

What the relationship between these centers and organized medicine should be is a bit difficult to spell out. For many clients there can well be an overlapping of concerns; for others, the psychologist will be providing services that are not salient to the interests or competence of medicine.

Since it is my thesis that the concept of disease is a broad one, with skills from many professions required for resolution, it would seem appropriate for psychologists to join alongside medicine in the health enterprise to render service to those whose needs are uniquely psychological (a view endorsed by Sarason and Gauzer 1968). This may be simpler to implement if the broad conception of health, rather than medicine, is used as the coordinating principle. Perhaps the most fruitful developments would come from a more vigorous redefinition, such as the one by Fuchs (1968):

". . . the biggest shortcoming of medical schools is indicated by their *name*. If they were to transform themselves into *schools of health*—with all that such a transformation implies for attitudes, objectives, personnel and curriculum—many of the. . . goals. . . would be closer to attainment.

A school of health would have the twin objectives of training personnel and advancing knowledge to meet the health needs of the community. It would define these needs broadly, would be concerned with the future as well as the present, and would meet health needs at various levels. . . The aim would be to provide a continuum of trained personnel to deal with a continuum of health problems. Some students would be ready for professional careers with less preparation than is currently required. Others might receive even more training than physicians do now.

. . . his yardstick of success would not be the number of cases in which he has personally been able to alter the course of events, but improvement in the health levels of the population that he and his colleagues serve." [10]

Who Gives the Treatment

The third element of the medical model, *who gives the treatment*, has also been in flux over these past few years. We have seen the explosion in medical knowledge, the sharpening of specialization in medical practice, the need for an entrance of a host of related professions and technical workers into the health field, and with all this a marked upswing in expectation of services for the general public. "In 1900, for every 100 physicians there were 60 health professionals trained in other fields, including 24 dentists, 1 registered nurse, 35 pharmacists, and others trained professionally. By 1960, the relative number of health professionals, other than physicians, had increased so that for every 100 physicians there were 371 other professionally trained health personnel."[13]

More recent data from the Allied Health Professions (Mase 1964) indicate that more than 13 workers join each physician in rendering health care. Health is indeed more than medication and physicians!

The categories of health worker are also expanding. A recent classification (Rutstein 1967) identified *other health professions* (nurses, medical social workers, pharmacists), *health vocations* (nurses aides, orderlies, laboratory assistants), *non medical employees in the health industry* (ambulance drivers, electricians, housekeeping staff), and *collaborative professions* (bio-chemists, medical economists, architects). Clinical psychologists are probably in the latter group.

Nor do we need to belabor well-known data on the limited availability of physicians—limited not only as a consequence of their numbers, but also because of their distribution and specialization. Thus, the National Commission on Community Health Services (1966) recommended that every individual have a personal physician, recognizing that trends in medicine are rendering such a goal ever less attainable. As contact between patient and physician grows more depersonalized, the hope some of us might have had that medicine would attend to the psychological and social aspects of disease grows more remote.

We are aware of some awakening movement toward equipping and orienting the physician to concern himself with the broad spectrum of disease through the training of family physicians, but it runs counter to the trend in American medicine, and we are guessing that other solutions may be needed.

It would seem reasonable to look to professions other than medicine to supply the personal contact that is now missing in health care. If we look to psychology, a report on psychology's manpower may be informative. Some 30,000 individuals believed to be psychologists (24,000 were APA members) were contacted for data. About 19,000 responded, and if we may extrapolate from their data to that of the total contacted population, the 36% who were clinical psychologists would provide a potential pool of 10,800 clinical psychologists in the United States. If we add the 11% in counseling and guidance, we have another 3,630. Combining the clinical and counseling and guidance psychologists, we would have a grand total of 14,430.

Assuming that each of these clinical and counseling psychologists would be available for collaboration with physicians for patient care services, we have a potential supply of one psychologist for each 20 physicians! And the future does not promise a better ratio since psychology is not increasing its production of professionals at any substantial rate.

It is clear that solutions for broadly based direct services to patients, involving biological, psychological, and social entities of disease, cannot be found in our present use of personnel. We shall have to seek new ways. If we should want to use psychologists to provide the psychological and social care we have described, it is unlikely that our current professionals, or those we are apt to produce over the next few years, will meet the needs.

The manpower picture I have outlined is not unfamiliar to most of us. The solutions lie in a number of areas: increasing the production of professionals, better utilization of high level skills of professionals, development of supporting personnel to aid existing professionals, development of specialized professionals to carry specific parts of the functions of the professional, *etc*. But recognizing the interprofessional character of health services and its breadth, we shall need to examine the system of delivery of services for duplication of effort, underutilization of skills, and nonfunctional restrictions on the exercise of skills. The system may need to be revamped to maximize the benefits of what personnel and abilities we can develop.

In the broad attack on disease—on maladaptation—we shall have to find the keys both to direct service to patients and clients and to intervention into the social system that is in part responsible for their maladjustments. This latter strategy provides the best hope for the future, as Bernard Bloom has eloquently pointed out in this book in his chapter on "Strategies for the Prevention of Mental Disorders."

Implied in this analysis of the health scene is the charge to psychology that its members will need to learn more about the social systems in which we live and the influence of these systems on individual maladaptation. Our continuing concern with intrapsychic phenomena will still be the figure against the ground of the social setting. We shall have to study figure and ground if we are to see the whole picture.

REFERENCES

1. Bloom, Bernard L., "Epidemiology for Preventive Services in Mental Health Programs," *Preventive Services in Mental Health Programs*, (Boulder: Western Interstate Commission for Higher Education, 1967).
2. Bloom, Bernard L., "Issues in Community Psychology and Preventive Mental Health," p. 14-15.
3. Boneau, Alan, "Psychology's Manpower," *Amer. Psychologist*, 1968, 23, 325-334.
4. Brown, Bertram S., and Long, S. Eugene, "Psychology and Community Mental Health: The Medical Muddle," *Amer. Psychologist*, 1968, 23, 335-341.
5. Colman, Douglas, "National Health Goals and Objectives," Speech presented at the National Health Forum, Chicago, March 20, 1967.
6. Cowen, Emory, Gardner, E. A., Zax, M., *Emergent Approaches to Mental Health.* (New York: Appleton, 1967).
7. Dubois, Rene, *Man Adapting*, (New Haven: Yale University Press, 1965).
8. Engel, George, "A Unified Concept of Health and Disease," *Perspect. Biol. and Med.*, 1960, 3, 459.

9. Engel, George, *Psychological Development in Health and Disease*, (Philadelphia: Saunders, 1962).

10. Fuchs, Victor R., "The Basic Forces Influencing Costs of Medical Care," *Federal Programs for the Development of Human Resources*, (Washington: US Government Printing Office, 1968) Vol. 2.

11. Gladston, Iago, *Beyond the Germ Theory*, (New York: Health Education Council, 1954).

12. Gordon, Ira, "Stimulation via Parent Education," *Children*, 16, 57-59.

13. *Health is a Community Affair*, Report of the National Commission on Community Health Services, (Cambridge, Mass.: Harvard University Press, 1966).

14. Hughes, Charles C., "Health and Well-being Values in the Perspective of Sociocultural Change," *Comparative Theories of Social Change*, (An.. Arbor: Foundation for Res. on Human Behav., 1966).

15. Magraw, Richard M., *Ferment in Medicine*, (Philadelphia: Saunders, 1966).

16. Mase, Darel, "Manpower Utilization for the Future," *Journal of Rehab.*, 1964.

17. May, Jacque, *The Ecology of Human Disease*, (New York: MD Publications, 1958).

18. Miller, George A., "Psychology as a Means of Promoting Human Welfare," *Amer. Psychologist*, 1969, 24, 1063-1075.

19. Rutstein, David D., *The Coming Revolution in Medicine*, (Cambridge, Mass.: The M.I.T. Press, 1967).

20. Sarason, Irwin and Gauzer, V. J., "Concerning the Medical Model," *Amer. Psychologist*, 1968, 23, 507-510.

21. Schaeffer, Morris and Hilleboe, H. E., "The Health Manpower Crisis: Cause or Symptom," *Amer. Journal Public Health*, 1967, 57, 6-14.

22. Sigerist, Henry, *Civilization and Disease*, (Phoenix Ed. 1943) (Chicago: University of Chicago Press, 1962).

23. Sprigle, Herbert, Van De Riet, Vernon and Van De Riet, Hani, "A Fresh Approach to Early Childhood Education." (Jacksonville, Florida: Authors, 1968).

24. Stainbrook, Edward, "Health and Disease and the Changing Social and Cultural Environment of Man," *Amer. Journal Public Health*, 1961, 51, 1005-1013.

25. Szasz, T. S., "The Myth of Mental Illness," *Amer. Psychologist*, 1960, 15, 113-118.

26. Szasz, T. S., "The Uses of Naming and the Origin of the Myth of Mental Illness," *Amer. Psychologist*, 1961, 16, 59-65.

27. Ullman, Leonard P. and Krasner, Leonard, *Case Studies in Behavior Modification*, (New York: Holt, Rinehart & Winston, 1965).

5: A Dimensional Strategy for Community Focused Mental Health Services*

Herbert Dörken

Our long-standing preoccupation with individual psychopathology and the possible intimate causes of disorder has had a restrictive and perverting influence on attempts to develop community mental health services. The definition of what constitutes abnormal behavior is largely sociocultural in nature. Further, the recognition of abnormality and the type of community action taken will have an enormous influence on the reported frequencies of various disorders and service demands, differing among social and cultural groups. If we are to meet both the needs and demands, it is through a social approach that we may gain long-term control and prevention of mental disorder.

Gorden, in discussing the epidemiology of alcoholism, adds another dimension to this perspective when he says, "No dread disease of man has ever been adequately controlled by attempts to treat the affected individual. Some progress can be made. There are ethical reasons for that approach. But if the objective is control of the condition in the population, the fundamental approach is through definition of the nature and extent of the problem and recognition of positive factors in prevention. A program based on treatment of the exaggerated illness is temporizing and with no promise of productive results. It is good clinical medicine, but poor public health." In the search for causes then, we must look to the ultimate causes of disorder: the living and working conditions of people, their homes, their economic insecurity, their social alienation, and their ignorance.

Most of us involved in community mental health services are really

*Based on presentation to the Western Missouri Mental Health Center, Kansas City, May 1967; The Corporation of Psychologists of the Province of Quebec, Montreal, March, 1968; Symposium on Community Mental Health, Loyola University, Chicago, May, 1968. The views expressed are those of the author and should in no way be construed as policy or practice of the Department.

thinking primarily of "local treatment services", when in my view, "community" is the key word. For a comprehensive community mental health service to become an effective agency, community involvement even to determination of policy is essential.

The comprehensive community mental health center has been advanced as a fundamental shift in strategy for handling mental disorders. Historically, and still too much today, the preferred solution has been to separate the mentally disordered person, to put him out of sight and mind, until, if he was lucky, he was returned to society. According to this old way, the community *abandoned* its responsibility for the mental patient to the distant mental hospital or left him to rely on private and confidential resources. According to the new way, the community *accepts* responsibility to develop coping resources and come to the aid of the citizen who is in trouble. The Center should not wait for serious psychological problems to develop and be referred or allow them to become more critical. Its programs for prevention, detection, and early intervention should involve it in many aspects of community life and in many institutions not normally considered as mental health agencies: schools, churches, playgrounds, welfare agencies, police, industry, and the courts. In this new pattern a person remains in his own community, often not leaving his home, close to family and friends and to a variety of agencies and professional people trying to help him.

This type of professional commitment reflects in part a new conception of mental disorder. The new concept questions the appropriateness of the term "illness" in this context, in spite of the recognition that much was gained from a humanitarian viewpoint in adopting the term. Mental disorders are in significant ways different from physical illnesses. Certainly, mental disorder is not the private misery of an individual. It often grows out of, and usually contributes to, the breakdown of normal sources of social support and understanding, especially within the family. It is not just an individual who has faltered. The social systems in which he is embedded through family, school, or job, through religious affiliation, or through friendship have failed to sustain him as an effective participant.

From this view of mental disorder, as rooted in social systems in which the troubled person participates, it follows that the objective of the center staff should be to help the various social systems of which the community is composed to function in ways which develop and sustain the effectiveness of individuals who take part in them, and to help those community systems regroup their forces to support the person who is in difficulty. The community is not just a catchment area from which patients are drawn. The task of the community mental health center goes far beyond that of purveying professional services to disordered people on a local basis. The more closely mental health centers become integrated with the lives and institutions of their community, the less the community can afford to turn over to mental health professionals its responsibility for guiding the center's policies. Admittedly, professional standards need to be established for the center by federal or state authorities, but goals and basic policies are a matter for local control. A broadly based, responsible board of informed leaders should help to insure that the center serves in deed, not just in name, as a focus for the community's varied efforts on behalf of the greater effectiveness and fulfillment of all its residents.

The dimensions of training, field research, program development, evaluation, consultation, and direct services need to be cast in a different perspective if we are to overcome basic errors in our strategy. Directionality in this schematic presentation is, from my point of view, both critical and atypical. In other words, we ordinarily start with "direct services" then provide "clinical consultation" and work up to "evaluation" and "program development" and so on. It should be quite the reverse. Moreover, in each dimension action should begin where community involvement can be comprehensive rather than at the point where it is only minimally feasible.

Training

Those responsible for the planning, administration, and financing of community mental health services have generally given only tangential, after-the-fact consideration to professional training. This is something that is dismissed with "the universities can do it" or "we'll leave it to

THE DIMENSIONS OF COMMUNITY MENTAL HEALTH SERVICES

(directionality is both critical and atypical)

Focus ——————————————— in ——————————————→ Depth

TRAINING

Career Orientation — Professional Training — Staff Development

FIELD RESEARCH

Problem Identity — Operational Research — Service Modification

PROGRAM DEVELOPMENT

Need Survey — Resource Development — Program Consolidation

EVALUATION

in

Accountability — Goals — Effectiveness

CONSULTATION

Establish Contacts — Develop Collaboration — Provide Coverage

DIRECT SERVICE

	Early Detection	—	Habilitation	—	Individual Treatment
	↑		↑		↑

Scope

Community Involvement	Comprehensive and Catalytic	Active but Limited	Minimal or Superficial

the big mental institutions, they have the patients and staff." It is as if, from our limited manpower pool, personnel, like moths, will continuously be lured to the new bright light of community mental health. But the need for personnel in state and non-community services has not decreased. Personnel drawn from hospital and clinical practice seldom have the experience or the perspective which leads them to involvement in community problems. They were not involved in community problems during their formative professional development. Their earlier ties have a potent residual effect attesting to the fact that behavior is shaped. Professional behavior is no exception. As we become older, behavior patterns crystallize, others describe it as "rigidity." Why not reach people during their formative years, not just the client, but also the staff? Personnel trained in the clinical tradition, despite attraction to novelty and new challenge, will, in the majority, continue to define community mental health services in terms of clinical services to individuals and will identify most readily with a hospital-illness orbit. This, in time, becomes the core. The community fades into the periphery. Such polarity, as it asserts itself, leads predictably to a compromise wherein the services must emanate. The intention of community service and involvement is then subverted. The representatives of the community can be put down in their efforts to determine the program and its direction with proclamations of medical responsibility. The individual in distress rather than the community becomes the unit of concern.

There is mounting evidence today that much of what we consider to be mental disorder is both socially determined and defined. The major faults of society lie not in its people but in its systems, and this premise is basic. Goffman's monograph points out the dehumanizing impact that our long-term mental hospitals have on patients. So too, the urban slum fosters an alienation process which precipitates dysfunctionality, leads to nowhere, and renders the individual powerless, locked out and without any opportunity for meaningful participation. Legislation which has supported programs such as the Economic Opportunities Act or the Poverty Movement seem to bear more directly on the mental health problems faced by communities then does the federal "comprehensive" Community Mental Health Centers Act.

By attending to social conditions, indeed, to the structure of society, we could focus on the seedbed of much that we classify as mental disorder. Now this conception views the community as the unit of concern. The community is the patient, not the individual. The official disorders within the community are the indices of its lack of well-being, and such factors as school drop-outs, divorce, illegitimate births, unemployment, bankruptcy, crime, and hospital commitments—their precursors and sequelae—are a recognized index of bio-psycho-social dysfunction. If we are serious in attacking the problem of mental disorder, is it most appropriate to give primary attention to the profound mental disorders of individuals? or try to rehabilitate those in difficulty? or intervene in crises as they arise? or seek to develop coping resources in the community? or seek to change adverse social conditions? The best strategy to enable prevention and control of what we term mental disorder would be in the exact reverse of the preceding sequence. But that would be opposite to the way we ordinarily proceed. To be sure, the emphasis on so-called illness and direct individual therapy is the backbone of most mental health professions and their training. It is, in the main, however, ill-suited to a sociological, ecological, even a public health approach. Adequate preparation will require a major shift in the content of training. The skills of the epidemiologist, market researcher, community planner, economist, educator, and politician have special relevance.

Each profession can wrangle about and evolve a suitable pattern of training, but before this dimension of training content can be crystallized, a new perspective on training is necessary. Community mental health planners have an inherent responsibility to consider the training and source of personnel if they are to meet the obligation to provide public service and solve mental health problems. Perhaps, this perspective is sharpened by detailing some underlying considerations:

1. The professional manpower pool can be augmented only by training.
2. There are no services without personnel.
3. The availability of manpower determines what services can be provided.
4. The pace of penetration of new professional services is directly related to the public sense of vacuum, need and relevance.

5. Established professions will resist a re-direction or re-definition of their services.
6. Services can be shaped by the control and direction of training.
7. The quality of service is related to the quality of staff.

In view of these operational facts, it can be argued that each community mental health service has an implicit responsibility to train personnel, and further, that the role of training is primary and essential to such programs if they are to be successful on a broad or sustained basis.

Ordinarily, when we talk of training, if we have staff on hand and an operating facility, we usually give first attention to staff development. We try, in other words, to tune up, hone, or sharpen those personnel that we already have. Perhaps we try to retread some of them: make nurses out of psychiatric technicians, psychiatrists out of physicians, social workers out of welfare aides, or psychologists out of counselors of psychometricians. Going back a step, we do give considerable attention to professional training but ordinarily in a manner divorced from the operating program. As for career orientation, *i.e.* getting the future citizen in his formative years and creating opportunities for his involvement in developing and continuing programs, it is a subject of much talk but rarely sustained action. This is the way it goes if we leave it to our basically self-interested professional staff. As for community involvement, it is minimal in regard to staff development.

In the established professional schools and universities, the community's involvement may be active, to be sure, though limited. But when we get down to the level of career orientation, we have the greatest possibility for a catalytic involvement of the community. The WICHE summer work-study program by the western states is an example of taking people in their early years in college and providing a summer orientation for them. They have two weeks of intensive orientation to mental health services, a six weeks' assignment to one of the operating mental health programs while affiliated with any one of the working disciplines of their choice, and then, a two weeks' windup at one of the state colleges in which they interchange experiences and gain a perspective on the total mental health program. This 10-week intensive career orientation draws heavily from among the brightest students and most of them find it a very exhilarating experience. This engagement with "real" life leaves many of the students with a new sense of participation and perspective. They react to it much like a short-term Peace Corps or Vista experience. Over one-half of the students later go on into one of the mental health professions or related careers.

Field Research

It is usual within mental health services to talk of ways of improving them. We try to modify our services, that is, according to the subjective judgment of those providing the service. Industry would undertake operational research, but mental health programs seldom do. Clinicians seem to avoid problem identification. They are too busy rendering services and going about their day to day tasks to stop and figure out why the services really exist in the first place. Even in the exception, when they try to determine the nature and extent of the problems needing attention, the solution proposed is too commonly just more of the same. If twenty sessions of psychotherapy haven't worked, many more are claimed to be needed—a testimonial to faith perhaps, but wanting in facts. What are the outcome data? Is the procedure specific to certain disorders or any disorder? Does it have differential effectiveness? Does it improve on base rate or expectancy data? Are these even known? Does it require highly involved and lengthy professional training to develop functional competence? How would it measure up in a cost-effectiveness study?

Ask professionals to engage in applied research, and there will be many clinical studies refining and modifying and expanding existing services. Even the mention of operational research is considered by many mental healthers as an infringement on their prerogatives and clinical skill. And the real problems of mental health at the community level? Find a respresentative group of citizens in the community, they will direct you to the problem and moreover, in relatively short time, can tell you whether your services have alleviated it.

Program Development

From research should come program development. In most communities there is a child guidance clinic and perhaps a mental hospital. Sometimes there are school psychological and mental health services, day care centers for the retarded, and related programs. You find bits and pieces of what might be a comprehensive mental health service scattered throughout a community. It is fashionable now to exercise the "continuity of caresmanship gambit" leading to consolidation of programs. Though sold on the notion of "continuity of care," it is, unfortunately, often a device for more unilateral professional control of all the programs which does not necessarily work to the advantage of any of them and makes community involvement less feasible. Many of these programs are best left decentralized rather than organized "from on high" and all given a similar stamp. They have a gatekeeper and control function.

The next phase which we may get into, but usually not sufficiently, is that of "resource development." We spend more of our time consolidating the programs that we have, rearranging them in various ways, clarifying their so called directions, but very little time actually going out into the community to develop *new* resources. More than that, if we develop the new resources, we tend to develop them from our perspective on the job. We don't develop them from the point of view of a need-survey. What the community really needs is quite often not what *we* perceive it needs. Most professionals don't really know their community. They live and work in an insular part of it and in these days of high mobility, many, if not most, are fairly recent arrivals.

Demographic and epidemiological studies are essential. The frequency and distribution of relevant bio-psycho-social disorders must be studied to pinpoint sources and the responsible systems. From these we are led to the real needs of the community, its real mental health problems. From this basis we can address ourselves to developing the resources to meet these needs, and once having the resources developed, *then* talk about consolidating or organizing the programs into some sequence of continuity. We typically proceed the other way around, which means that we are terribly busy providing services, not ncessarily relevant to community mental health needs, and seldom solving any of the inherent problems.

Evaluation

Program evaluation is also a very sensitive issue to professional people. Clinicians who talk about the effectiveness of their programs are usually quite defensive about them, and more so since Eysenck published his work on the effectiveness of out-patient psychotherapy. Isn't it remarkable how many patient groups, untreated, given only custody or treated by different professional disciplines, or treated by many different methods all seem to show about a 70% recovery rate! Perhaps the treatment is of more benefit to the professionals than to the clients involved. Outcome data, however, will show that actually we do have some services that are symptom-specific or disorder-specific and where we can actually improve upon the natural baserate of expectancy. The behavior modification techniques based on learning theory and conditioning are showing great promise. Their greater amenability to measurement is alone an overwhelming advantage. Together with computer facilities, the means to undertake program evaluation is now at hand. We can then, if we will, evaluate the effectiveness of our current programs for our current client population, but I believe it is even more important to go back a step and specify our goals. It is more logical to make program goals explicit first and then evaluate the effectivenss of services in relation to them rather than simply study what we are doing.

Even more basic is the concept of accountability. Who is held accountable and for what? This is an issue that professional people in the mental health services—universities too—have managed to avoid very neatly. But those of us involved with the public or the public's representatives in the legislature are increasingly held to an accountability. If you go before a Ways and Means Committee and claim you need certain dollars or personnel or authority to do a job, they assume that if they provide it, you are going to deliver. And next year or at the next session they are going to want to know what you accomplished. Did you meet the goals; to what extent and how? And if not, why not? Is the coverage better, and is there evidence within the community that services have improved or the need has diminished? How many of us providing direct mental health services hold ourselves accountable to anybody, either for time or for a range of coverage of our services, or for the effectiveness of them? This is a dimension that will come increasingly to public attention as state and federal governments become involved in a range of mental health services, in contrast to operating isolated institutions. This is particularly true when they become prepaid services as in national health insurance or medicare. Cost accounting procedures have already had a notable impact on hospital services and when cost effectiveness becomes the guideline, clinicians will undergo a revolution. Why the squeeze? The public at large is now involved.

The more there is community involvement and representation in contrast to strictly professional determination, control and delivery of services, the broader will be their base of support. They will be more widely recognized within the community. This factor of visibility carries an inherent self-correcting mechanism, since it is more feasible to acclaim or criticize that which is known. The services are no longer a private and confidential endeavor of several professions with a fraction of the population. The services are public—they are to the community. Viewed along a dimension from indirect to direct services, it is the indirect services which carry greater visibility.

Consultation

As for consultation, we usually think first of clinical consultation which is a means of extending our current clinical services just a little further, making a somewhat more efficient use of limited professional expertise. But that doesn't necessarily involve us in any real collaborative arrangement. The tactic is to come in, give advice and then bow out. After all, *you* do it, it's *your* case" (or your problem). In program consultation we have the convenient rationale that the client or the agency "has to reach its own decisions," a sort of transfer of the psychotherapeutic model to consultation. But a collaboration in which both parties as co-participants are to be held responsible for the outcome usually finds them gun-shy.

We could of course take the initiative in extending consultative services to the community by "establishing contacts." How many community mental health services are really trying to penetrate into the community? Clinicians typically sit in their offices and wait for referrals to come in. They are very concerned about how to have an open or closed referral system, or what is an appropriate source, or how to develop a valid set of screening devices. But to go to the root source, to know the circumstances that people come from or why, that's something most fail to do. One of the early programs of this nature was the Montefiore Hospital in the Bronx, with services organized on a census tract basis. The urbanite professional—and there are a few others—will typically offer the excuse that in rural settings, where communities are not very complex, they can be easily sized up, but in a big city there is too much transition, too many people and too few services. Do you simply avoid a problem? Each staff member can be held responsible for a specific section or census tract. He must find out what's behind every door. In that way he really comes to know the living conditions of the people there, who lives there, what resources exist in that area and what liabilities it has from the standpoint of the city mental health program. Once the contacts have been established and you know what your're really dealing with in terms of social structure and problems, you have a basis from which to develop collaboration among all the interested parties. From this effective coverage evolves, not the other way around.

Direct Service

Most of the mental health professionals are involved in individual treatment. When service demands become excessive, the first resort is usually to group psychotherapy. Here, too, the selection for group experience can become quite sophisticated. But in many cases what is probably needed is not treatment, but "habilitation." This is in essence shaping the behavior and the conditions of people such that they can adapt to their circumstances or adapt their circumstances to them. Such human or social engineering—the counseling or environmental manipulation approaches—though usually dismissed by clinicians, carry the promise of relevance and should be attempted before we try actual "treatment." If a simple or straightforward solution is available, why be complex? Token economy programs applied to the chronic schizophrenic also illustrate the habilitation concept.

The behavior to be shaped is operationally defined and change is then more amenable to measurement. Constructive and self responsible behavior is outlined and as it occurs is rewarded. These programs do not simply reach the individual or carry meaning for him; they create a relevant social system in which constructive behavior is encouraged. Preoccupation with intrapsychic conflicts is minimized, while effective participation and accomplishment are maximized.

But before treatment or habilitation, should we not be concerned with case finding or the early detection of disorders within the community? We have possibilities here that we lightly overlook, though citizen participation would be more effective at this level. Should it take a full blown psychosis to mobilize action?

Conclusion

If we are to have community focused mental health services, we ought to start at the level where community action is most natural and work over to the professional services rather than the reverse. Further, our efforts should proceed from a training, to research, to program development orientation rather than the usual preoccupation with clinical services and consultation.

6: Evaluation in Community Mental Health

J. Wilbert Edgerton

Evaluation in community mental health is a particularly timely subject for the decade of the 1970's in the United States. If we dare to be optimistic, the stage may be set for the heavy drain on our resources, due to the war in Vietnam, to be considerably reduced, and once again we can turn our monies and attention to our massive domestic problems, including community mental health. We have only begun to develop the "bold new approach" to mental health problems envisaged in the Community Mental Centers Act of 1963 (Public Law 88-164), and as amended in 1965 (Public Law 89-105). We are poised, as it were, between this start and what promises to become a large and very expensive program in the coming years. Evaluation of our methods in community mental health should be re-emphasized and widely instituted as a measure to assure the best possible program investment before the patterns are irrevocably set. Our present opportunity is reminiscent of the situation confronting the long-ago motorist on the midwestern plains who came to a sign which read, "Choose your ruts, you'll be in them for the next 50 miles." We may now be choosing our community mental health program patterns for the next fifty years, and if so, we should not only know what we are doing but have systems for deriving valid data and the means for modifying those programs long before the decade of the 2020's. Admittedly there is optimism here, for the large public mental hospital system, with all its contributions and its evils, has been with us more than a century.

Evaluation is timely also because we are moving to a philosophy which says that good mental health is a right, not just a privilege, and to implement that ideal we say that our community mental health programs shall be available financially and be accessible geographically to *all* the people. We can no longer afford, financially or morally, the luxury of developing just any mental health program with the idea that it will be a contribution. We must have a means for making rational choices as to the most effective range of community services for the mental health needs of the people. In addition, the people have the right to knowledge as to the return-rate on their program investment. Evaluation is the means through which the appointed stewards of program resources account for their trust.

The sheer extensiveness of recent programs designed to eliminate social, economic, educational, health and mental health deficits and deprivation forces some determination of program effectiveness, and particularly if continued support is to be forthcoming. The needs have been so compelling that we have been willing to accept many new programs on faith. But we are entering an era of increasing emphasis on solving social problems through planned action which must be based on existing and advancing knowledge.

More and more, mental health problems are seen as affecting the whole community and not just those families whose members have required remedial assistance. Nor are mental health problems only the concern of those traditional mental health professions of psychiatry, clinical psychology, psychiatric social work, and psychiatric and mental health nursing. Rather, changes at the community level are mandatory and must involve the cooperation of official and voluntary agencies, the professionals and the citizen groups. Programs of prevention of disorder and coordination and integration of services, the consequence of changes in the social environment, must supplant programs consisting largely of treatment and rehabilitation. Evaluation of such programs will necessarily reflect changed objectives and different criteria of effectiveness.[20]

Two recent examples of official support of evaluation will help to further underline the timeliness and attest to the favorable climate for evaluation in community mental health. The Community Mental Health Centers Act of 1963, and as amended in 1965, together with the regulations governing their implemenation, names "research and evaluation" as one element of the program of adequate services of the comprehensive mental health center and provides Federal support for construction of facilities and for professional and technical personnel for research and evaluation activities (P.L. 88-164; P.L. 89-105; P.L. 88-164: Regulations; P.L. 89-105: Regulations). The nature of the research and evaluation program was described as "research in mental illness, epidemiological studies of incidence and distribution of mental illness in the community, and evaluation of the treatment procedures and programing of the center."[10]

The other example is the "Comprehensive Health Planning and Public Health Service Amendments of 1966" (P.L. 89-749), and their extension in the "Partnership for Health Amendment of 1967" (P.L. 90-174). These acts authorize extensive amounts of money for assisting states to establish and maintain comprehensive public health services (P.L. 89-749, p. 4) and for project grants for developing health services in a limited geographic area; to stimulate innovations in providing health services; and to finance studies, demonstrations, or training for developing new methods or improving present methods of providing health services (P.L. 90-174, p. 2). Fifteen percent of the money for comprehensive public health services must go to mental health programs (P.L. 89-749, p. 5) and at least seventy percent must be available only for services in the communites of the states (P.L. 90-174, p. 2). The issue here is the fact that up to one percent of the funds under the two aspects of this program are available to the Secretary of Health, Education, and Welfare for program evaluation (P.L. 90-174, p. 8). Under present authorization this means $3,650,000 could be utilized by the Secretary for program evaluation by June 30, 1970. Another section of the acts adds another $130,000 for program evaluation (P.L. 90-174, p. 2). The corresponding available amounts as specified for community mental health program evaluation would be $285,000.

In sum, public policy as reflected in a community-level program focus, responding to the needs of all the people, the growing concern of professionals in the mental health field, and of the citizenry itself, together provide a mandate for evaluation in community mental health which cannot be comfortably ignored.

Psychologists have contributed heavily to research in the mental health field, disproportionately more than their sheer numbers have warranted. This is a tribute to their interests, but is undoubtedly also a reflection of their training in scientific methods of investigation. Too, they have been attracted by the availability of mental health research funds from many sources. So it is reasonable to expect psychologists to continue their involvement with the mental health research endeavor even as community programs proliferate, even *because* they proliferate, and there is coincidental interest to pursue community investigations both as citizens and as scientist-professionals. If specific encouragement from their fellows is needed, it has been recorded in numerous places. The Joint Commission on Mental Illness and Health (Joint Commission, p. XXII) recommended that funds for research in the mental health field be provided at the rate of two and one-half percent of patient service budgets. To name only one other, the position paper of the American Psychological Association on the mental health center called for an explicit portion of the budget of the community mental health center to be devoted to program evaluation (Smith & Hobbs, 1966, p. 21) in order that "worthy approaches be retained and refined, ineffective ones dropped."[25] The recommendation was that "every center should devote between 5% and 10% of its budget to program evaluation and research."[25]

Having made the case for the timeliness, the efficacy, and the necessity for evaluation in community mental health, and predicted the continuing involvement of psychologists with the mental health reserach and evaluation enterprise, it remains to examine some of the problems in evaluation, the role of the psychologist in carrying it out, and the strategies and challenges confronting him.

The Problem of Evaluation

Evaluation is constantly with us, even in community mental health. We begin with the value that it is good to have good mental health. In support of this value, we set as a goal the provision of resources through which our citizens can achieve it. This allocation of resources frequently takes the form of treatment services designed to restore health or provide rehabilitation. At a very informal and inexplicit level, we make the judgment that to have these treatment services is good.

Other communities have them, they are recommended by the National Institute of Mental Health, so we should have them in our community. Of course, this level of evaluative judgement says nothing about whether the treatment services are really restoring people to good mental health, or whether the professional staff or the community sponsors are having their expectations met or are getting their money's worth. Evaluation means making a judgment and implies that there are standards against which judgments may be made. Obviously the standards may be implicit or explicit, so that evaluations may vary from the impressionistic and relatively informal to the most systematic and quantitative. In either case the evaluation must be made against internal criteria: Is the treatment program accomplishing what was set for it to do? Or it must be made against external criteria: How does it compare with other such efforts? With national standards? How is it perceived by a panel of experts? Are the results reflected in objective community data, such as changes in admission rates?

This is to emphasize that there are levels of evaluation. Another way to illustrate this is through the following set of questions:

1. Does the population know of the available resources?
2. Knowing the availability of the resources, are the people then in contact with them?
3. If the people are in contact with the resources, how long are they in contact? What is the extent of their use of the resources?
4. What is the impact of the resources (services) at both the individual and community levels?[7]

The psychologist should be cognizant of the informal, day-to-day, subjective evaluations that occur in community mental health as well as of the relatively simple to complex levels of evaluation.The stance here will be that he can contribute to the collection of more reliable information at any level in spite of a number of problems which must be taken into account.

A distinction is frequently made between research and evaluation (NIMH, 1955; Jackson, 1967; James, 1962). Research is considered to be carried out in order to discover new knowledge for its own sake and independent of its utility. Evaluation, on the other hand, is conducted in order to determine the degree of success in reaching predetermined objectives. Evaluations is concerned with accomplishment or with the assessment of a technique utilized in the service of the goals of accomplishment (MacMahon, Pugh, & Hutchison, 1961). Its purpose is to collect information upon which improved methods or techniques or whole programs can be based. It should be clear, however, that both research and evaluation require testable hypotheses, valid and reliable measuring devices or procedures, precision in design, adequate controls, and definable criteria. It is acknowledged, though, that in evaluation efforts in mental health, the experimental conditions of the laboratory rarely prevail, and never in mental health programs in the community. Inference here is limited in its generality because of the problems of control in community studies, even though the independent variable inputs do make a significant difference in the dependent variable outcomes.

A further characteristic of evaluation research is that decisions as to resource allocation or program change are likely to hinge on its outcomes. At least that is hopefully possible in those enlightened program endeavors in which administrators and evaluators are in effective communication.

So far evaluation efforts have been devoted largely to therapeutic techniques for specific individual pathological conditions, and the literature abounds with reports of these activities. Other evaluations have concerned some individual agency or program practice. Despite the criterion problem in therapeutic effectiveness, these endeavors have contributed to the evolution of treatment methods and mental health program development through the years but have not shown their adaptability, application, or transferability to the problems of mental health in the total community (Freeman & Sherwood, 1965; Greving, 1957).

Psychologists must share with the other professional disciplines the responsibility for this state of affairs. But the time has come when concerted attention must be given to the "reciprocal relationships between individuals and the social systems which constitute the community context."[2] The complex social, economic, and political interdependence brought on by our increasing urbanism has increased the vulnerability of the individual to risks which take away his opportunities and freedom to realize his maximum potential. In turn, this results in stresses that are reflected in poor mental health or at minimum, in the loss of opportunity to enhance mental health.

To prevent or ameliorate these stresses or to render individuals less vulnerable will require interventions not administered separately to the social, economic, or political environmental systems. Rather, the interventions must be applicable to any or all of these systems at the point of their dynamically integrated impact, and the means for evaluating their effectiveness must be available or invented particularly. Whole community populations, or diverse population subgroups, more and more must be the object of concern if progress is to be made in solving the problems of community mental health—the problems of human living. Therefore, not only should continuing efforts be devoted to refining treatment, or rehabilitative interventions directed at individuals, but it is imperative that conceptual models be perfected which can provide systematic approaches to, and valid information about, the effects of such interventions at the environmental systems level on population aggregates. Prominent devices already in use include the epidemiological, the systems analysis, and the ecological models. Modified versions of these have also been put to use and further combinations and elaborations are in order.

Another order of problem in evaluation in community mental health is the nature of the variable with which we must at some time be concerned. The quality in which we are interested, mental health, exists as a continuous variable, not in discrete categories (Glidewell & Domke, 1957). Mental health is not a quality that is present or absent; it exists in degrees of more or less. If we assess the mental health of an individual, we are making judgments as to the degree of its existence in comparison with some standard, some criterion. Or if we look at the impairment of mental health we are judging its degree of existence against some standard. The exact relationship between mental health and the impairment of mental health, or mental disorder, has not been specified. Whether they vary inversely, or even along the same continuum, has not been established. Mental health and mental disorder never exist in observable absolute quantities because we have not been able to specify an end point at which they are non-existent from which to measure nor establish units of direct measure. So we can only describe changes in them.

The presence of mental health or mental disorder as qualities is inferred and usually described in terms of observable behaviors which have been defined as indicative of health or disorder. Changes in these behaviors then imply changes in mental health or mental disorder. The task of the mental health evaluator is to infer the amount or nature of the changes in behavior induced by deliberate environmental interventions. This task is of an order of greater complexity than if the quality under consideration existed in discrete categories of presence or absence, as in the communicable diseases.

That behavior is a function of the situation in which it occurs, as well as of the genetic endowment of the behaver, is not disputed anymore. That changing the situation results in a change in behavior is of the order of a truism for psychologists. But now there is ample evidence that mental patients, for example, subjected to the anonymous routinized schedule of long-term hospitalization, suffer from effects beyond those directly associated with their disorders themselves. The patient's normal social relationships are disrupted to be replaced by various forms of social disability (A.P.H.A., 1962). Clearly this is a response to the chronic ward social system, and has shown its amenableness to change through a number of programs designed to normalize the treatment experience—open hospitals, "total push," milieu therapy, remotivation, family care, and others. Changing the social system is reflected in changed behavior. Appropriate interventions in the social system lead to improvement in mental health or reductions in disorder or impairment.

Whether in a dyad, a family, an institution, or the multiple social systems of the community—the social, the economic, and political as well as health care systems—a person's individual behavior reflects the interacting social forces. The evaluator may focus on any of the systems. He may be interested in the effectiveness of a therapeutic method on an individual, and he must concern himself with the effects on whole groups of people of community level interventions, such as mental health programs. In case of a prevention program his population may be a particularly susceptible group of persons. In case of a treatment program, it may be a group of people with a particular illness or a group of illnesses.[17] Because the health system is interlocked with the social, economic, and political systems, it may be necessary to intervene in all systems at once, which adds greatly to the complexity of the task of evaluation in community mental health.

The Psychologist as Evaluator

Psychologists have knowledge and competencies which can be turned to community mental health research and program evaluation. They know something of research design, control methods, criterion definitions and statistical and measurement requirements. However, they must learn the community orientation—how to apply these research principles to social-cultural contexts. Their traditions equip them for experimental observation where, though the variables are vastly complex, valid criteria and control methods are easier to come by. Their training is much less likely to have provided experience in operations or systems research involved with comparisons of groups, or repeated observations over time with a given cohort, or with a changing community context. They are not so accustomed to observing patterns of development or correlated patterns of behavior and environmental events in natural settings. The task of inferring that a given intervention does what it is designed to do is indeed causally related to changes in behavior of individuals or groups, is more difficult than in the usual experimental laboratory research and may strain the ambiguity-tolerances of those investigators whose comfort derives from less tenuous certitudes. Community mental health evaluative research may be considered to be an observational science in contrast to an experimental laboratory research, and may strain the ambiguity-psychologists adapt to this tentative "science"? Can they live with situations which require treating some people in need and not others in order to further our knowledge? How about the difficulties in trying to match cities or towns or counties? Certainly psychologists have some obligation to contribute to the development, refinement, and extension of methods of evaluative research and some obligation to assist in the erection of a scientific base for the planned interventions into the community systems designed to raise the level of mental health.

Another attribute of psychologists which should qualify them to participate in evaluative research in the community is their broad orientation to human behavior. That is to say that they are accustomed to observing behavior across the total spectrum of normal to abnormal, of well to sick, of serene to disturbed, of mature to immature, of adult to child, crosssectional or developmentally throughout the total life span. They have looked at behavior comparatively from protozoa to mammals, and some have made intercultural comparisons. They have looked at solitary behavior, cooperative and competitive behavior in dyads, in triads, and behavior in larger small groups. They are not by any means as accustomed to predicting and controlling the behavior of large groups collectively occupying a given geographic locus. But the fact that psychologists have not been oriented only to deviant behavior perhaps gives them a more valid perspective from which to apply their evaluative and assessment procedures to the effects of the whole gamut of environmental forces on human behavior and on mental health. To this point their principal professional colleagues in the mental health field have been predominantly occupied with individual pathological behavior as rooted in the bio-medical tradition. Such occupation has led to a primary investment in the treatment and rehabilitation of the moderately and severely mentally ill. Psychologists, however, with interest in normal development, and even the promotion of mental health, have given some attention to preventive program activity—strengthening individuals to withstand environmental stress, or teaching significant people how to modify or to divert potentially damaging environmental forces so as to protect the individual. Preventive program evaluation is undoubtedly the most difficult to carry out, but by the same token should have a high priority in community mental health.

Because of his training and investment in methods of investigation, it may be posited that the psychologist is the logical one of the more traditional mental health disciplines to move toward community mental health program evaluation. The clinical psychologist, skilled in individual assessment, whose appreciation of intra-psychic functioning allows him to reliably predict behavior in response to environmental forces, is qualified for individual assessment procedures involved in evaluation, particularly therapeutic interventions. This is but a step away from assessment of behaviors correlated with the environmental events of the larger social, economic, or political systems. He can also appreciate the special difficulties of criterion definition and measurement procedures, as well as inter-judge or inter-investigator agreement. The principles are the same as he moves from assessment of individual response to environmental interventions, to assessment of the response of groups of individuals to environmental interventions at the social systems level. It's that the arena is greatly enlarged, and the interventions frequently more diffuse and less specific in their effects than, for example, in the case of testing the effects of a new drug on individual behavior. But in both instances the focus is a dynamic, changing, on-going system.

Other Important Skills and Evaluation Strategies

Even so, it will be necessary for the clinical psychologist-turned-community psychologist-evaluator to have at least a practical knowledge of a wide range of methods, or at least to be able to draw on the knowledge and techniques of his fellow psychologists and colleagues from other professions. This means considerable effort devoted to the logistics of intercommunication with sociologists, social psychologists, anthropologists, epidemiologists, biostatisticians, political scientists, city planners, program administrators, public health professionals, social psychiatrists, economists, and perhaps the consulting philosopher. It is presumed that he has already learned to communicate with the other professionals of his clinical world—the psychiatrist, the social worker, the psychiatric or mental health nurse, the special teacher, and the adjunctive therapists. He not only stands to learn from all of these people, but they are necessary to the evaluation processes if indeed he hopes to be an evaluator of a total program. Necessary to him, too, is the skill of communicating with the consumers of program services—the clients or patients, and the other mental health service-givers in the community (the teacher, the welfare worker, the lawyer, the minister, the judge, the policeman, the rehabilitation counselor, the agency administrator, the physician, the home demonstration or agricultural extension worker, and others). Information from these people and from the general citizen in the community will provide a basis for making judgments about program effectiveness and hopefully lead to a more efficient allocation of material and human resources.

It should go without saying that the evaluator should have a thorough grounding in the principles and methods of evaluation design in community mental health. But added to this should be some knowledge of multivariate data analysis techniques which are feasible in this age of the computer. Demographic and other social factors data have a way of varying together, or seemingly so, and sensible systems interventions can be devised more specifically with this kind of information. Population sampling techniques will be required, for in working with defined geographic areas, it will be necessary to assure representativeness. Assessment of whole population groups will be rarely possible in view of the cost in time, money, and manpower. It has already been indicated that the methods of systems analysis, epidemiology, and ecological analysis are necessary for the complex interactions which are the focus here. They can tell us what effective interventions might be and where and when to apply them for maximum benefit. If systematic cost-benefit data are ever to be available in community mental health programs, they will have to come through the systems approach or one of its variants. Evaluators must do their share in devising valid measures of input and output units for the actualizing of this conceptual ordering of events and data. Indeed the responsibility for design that permits the specification of the relationship between input variables and goals must be theirs.

This brings up two related ideas in evaluation strategy. One is the importance of firsthand experiential contact of the evaluator with the procedures or program being evaluated. The evaluator must know exactly what actions are being carried out in order to specify appropriate data and to devise a means of collecting them. Ideally, he will have a voice in the decision about what actions are being carried out in order to meet the objectives, which he also had a part in formulating in the first place. There is no problem with this issue if the program practitioner is doing the evaluation; if the latter is the case, strategies for assuring objectivity must be employed. In any case there must be close association between the program practitioner and the evaluator in order to have collaborative resolution of differences for any part of the total procedure. Another advantage of this association is the opportunity it provides for communicating the findings of the evaluation procedure to the crucial person for program change and for re-allocation of resources. All too frequently these two people live in splendid isolation from each other, friendly, each respecting the other, but with findings not utilized in improved program effectiveness.

The other of the two related ideas in evaluation strategy noted above is the importance of building evaluation into all program practices from their inception. Not only does this permit tailoring practice and evaluation procedures to each other, but it cultivates and facilitates an evaluative or critical investigative attitude within the program staff members. It helps to establish budget policies that legitimize evaluation along with service, not leaving it to the whims of fortune or the wiles of some penny-wise budget officer. It saves money in the long run, for program activities with no pay-off can be eliminated and resources can be allocated more effectively. In fact, built-in continuous evaluation allows for appropriate intermediate changes on the way to the overall goals, the bases for which would not otherwise become apparent. It also can demonstrate the importance of doing even simple evaluations that give some information on outcomes, and this is very important for a staff that may stand in awe of the complicated procedures of evaluation, not to mention the fear of being on trial in program performance. Such fears, incidentally, emphasize the importance of eliciting staff cooperation and establishing confidence in the evaluators in order that staff roles in data collection, if any, will be fulfilled. Initiating change as a result of the findings of evaluation procedures will also be vastly facilitated by providing information to staff members at appropriate times and including them in the decision processes for implementation.

An aspect of evaluation to be borne in mind is that different investors in the community mental health enterprise may have different goals, and hence expect different outcomes. Hence, the evaluator will be

faced with the problem of different sets of criteria of success for the
many publics interested in his findings. He is fortunate indeed if in
meeting the expectations of one public he is able to meet the
expectations of all. The community which provides the services may be
content to know that the services are there, purely on the judgment
that it is an acceptable thing to do. But it may want some evidence that
it is getting its money's worth, in which case a statistical report of
services may suffice. The sponsoring community board members may
want still another kind of evidence that their efforts are paying off.
They may require data on rate of improvement if it is a treatment
service. The program staff may have goals of program development that
include far less treatment services, for example, than envisioned by the
other professional people in the community. Obviously the evaluator
would be involved with priorities somewhat at variance with each other,
and his procedures would in turn be affected. Client or patient goals
might require less of the evaluator's efforts in providing data, but
clearly that group is one of the publics with which he would be
concerned. So his evaluation may range all the way from simple
program description to the most sophisticated analysis of program
effectiveness, depending on the particular public. He wants to
determine whether the results coincide with goals of each investment
group. In some instances he may judge program performance and
results against outside criteria. The evaluator's total program evaluation
may require a system of continuous monitoring of criterion variables at
several levels from the treatment case level, to the agency functioning
level, to the community system level. And he, himself, may be yet
another one of his publics.

Another timely approach to evaluation in community mental health
is that of the role functions of the many varieties of professional,
technical, non-professional and supportive personnel who man the
comprehensive programs. It is not enough to analyze the written job
descriptions on which the people were hired. Data must be gathered on
what they actually do. It is already apparent that the usual roles and
distinctive functioning of the collaborating mental health disciplines
have become somewhat blurred through the application of the
criterion of competence (Joint Commission, p. 248; Yolles, 1966, p.

40), and each may be called upon to perform in ways not formally prescribed. New roles are being created and their contributions need to be understood. Clinical psychologists, for example, are developing screening instruments, conducting research on staff procedures and outcomes, doing operations research, and mounting consultation and prevention programs. Can the psychologist, as practitioner, move freely in the inpatient, outpatient, and emergency services, and consultation and education program elements of the comprehensive mental health center? Can he be attuned to the community forces and resources and understand the means and processes for effecting appropriate changes in the community, or even in his agency? Is he skilled in group development and group therapy techniques, and can he assist in the management of the therapeutic milieu? Can he, as an evaluator, make the assessments for program change that he, as a psychologist, will carry out? Is he an observer who can participate in the process he observes? These are some of the role changes to be expected, and it is obvious that systematic evaluation of the use of human resources in relation to program results is central to the whole evaluative effort. Innovative utilization of manpower is an imperative, but it must be consonant with explicit goals.

The Challenge and the Opportunity

In the foregoing sections, emphasis has been given to the necessity for evaluation in community mental health, to a number of the problems encountered, and the rationale for and some of the advantages offered by psychologists as evaluators. Attention was also given to some of the important strategies and necessary skills for evaluation studies.

It may be somewhat anticlimactic to indicate that there remains a host of unsolved problems in evaluation in community mental health. The central one is the objectification and standardization of criteria for judging change in mental health or disorder status. An allied problem is the lack of objective methods for characterizing the disability of patients. Valid data on the degree of impairment and of psychosocial changes in patients are needed to facilitate comparisons of groups from different communities and for criterion measures on the effects of programs of intervention (Kramer, Pollock, Locke, & Bahn, 1961). A notable attempt in this direction are the Katz Adjustment Scales which cover psychiatric symptoms and social behaviors, in addition to social role performance, recreation and free time activities, and relatives' expectations and satisfaction with the patient's performance (Katz & Lyerly, 1963). The Scales give valid measures of behavior at various levels of adjustment in and out of the hospital and differentiate between normals and hospitalized, normals and day center patients, and day center and hospitalized patients. The Scales have been used in getting an estimate of the prevalence rate of untreated disorder in a general population (Hogarty, et. al., 1967). Although numerous studies have attempted to establish this ratio, it still remains one of the important challenges to mental health program evaluation when applied to a whole community. A related problem is the lack of success in devising valid instruments for assessing the mental health of those people without impairment.

Psychologists may be able to help establish wider and more profitable usage of psychiatric case registers, from which it is possible to establish unduplicated counts of individuals for computation of rates of admission to psychiatric care in a given area. This is but one of the devices in a system of information-gathering on total populations which is so greatly needed for ordering the inputs into, and outputs from, the community system. Related to this, it has been suggested that another useful device would be a psycho-social register which would establish standard reporting for all community agencies and permit systematic assessment of psycho-social-cultural factors as they relate to mental disorder (Sata, 1967, p. 354). It would help locate the disorder in high risk groups and facilitate attention to other factors related to the assessment of mental health. We do need to be sensitive to data which have relevance to the consequences of interventions in the social system, other than demographic and resource utilization in the conventional sense.

Another front in need of attention from the psychologist-evaluator is that of cost-benefit analysis or cost-effectiveness. These are terms and procedures borrowed from economists. It seems clear that progress here will require a systems analysis approach, and this in turn will require considerable ingenuity with the techniques of inferential statistics and research design in comparing predetermined objectives and observable outcomes. An elegant treatment of some of these issues may be found in a paper by Levy, Herzog, and Slotkin (1966). Closely related to cost-effectiveness ideas is the use of "planning-programing-budgeting systems" (PPBS, Novick, 1965). The main features of this approach, which mandates evaluative studies, include written plans, alternate choices for accomplishing goals, and cost-benefit analyses of the choices. Clearly this is another attempt to manage data relating need to resources in such a way as to delineate profitable and effective interventions.

We have been wont to do program evaluations to show that a given activity in which we are invested is worthwhile. It is rare that accounts of our program failures find their way into print. It is probably true that we learn equally as much from our failures as our successes. The plea here is for really critical evaluation which looks at the impact of our system interventions on individual people and the community. No amount of the measurement of program effort will do.

In line with really critical evaluation is the need to look at the unexpected outcomes and the possible dangerous or beneficial side effects of the really good accomplishment of program goals. What, for example, will be the ultimate effect on the level of pathology in the community when more and more schizophrenics live there, marry, and procreate? What other measures will then be necessary? Hopefully, interventions will be devised which lower the incidence of disorder. Can we also expect shorter durations of illness and milder disability? Interventions which affect mental health are likely also to affect physical health. Examples of unintended side effects, harmful and beneficial, abound in other contexts, but the challenge here is to use as much perspective as possible and to anticipate as broadly as possible in order not only to specify the intended effects, but to be alert to changes in other parts of the system or sub-system.

All of these problems offer a formidable challenge to the imagination, creativity, and working energies of psychologists who would improve the opportunities for good mental health and self-actualization for all.

There is also the specific challenge of demonstrating the effectiveness of wide-scale consultation efforts in community mental health—that method so heralded as the first officially mandated preventive program effort in the field.

With persistent attack, head-on, or in strategic flanking approaches, these challenges can be converted into opportunities.

REFERENCES

1. American Public Health Association, Program Area Committee on Mental Health. *Mental Disorders: A Guide to Control Methods.* (New York, N. Y.: APHA, 1962) Chapter 1, 1-22.
2. By-Laws, Division of Community Psychology, American Psychological Association. Newsletter, 1967, 1, No. 1.
3. *Community Mental Health Centers Act of 1963, Title II, Public Law 88-164: Regulations.* Reprinted from the Federal Register, May 6, 1964.
4. *Comprehensive Health Planning and Public Health Services Amendments of 1966.* Public Law 89-749, 89th Congress, (Washington, D. C.: Government Printing Office, 1966).
5. Freeman, H., and Sherwood, C., "Research in Large-scale Intervention Programs," *The Journal of Social Issues, 1965,* 21, 11-28.
6. Glidewell, J., *Personal Communication,* 1968.
7. Glidewell, J., and Domke, H., "Health Department Research in Community Mental Health," paper presented to annual meeting of American Public Health Association, Cleveland, November, 1957.
8. Greving, F. T., "Practical Issues in Evaluating Community Mental Health Services," Conference of Chief Social Workers from State Mental Health Programs, Philadelphia, May, 1957.
9. Hogarty, G., Katz, M., and Lowery, H., "Identifying Candidates from a Normal Population for a Community Mental Health Program." Russell R. Monroe, Gerald O. Klee, and Eugene B. Brody (Eds.), *Psychiatric Epidemiology and Mental Health Planning.* (Washington, D. C.: American Psychiatric Association, 1967) 220-234.
10. House of Representatives Report No. 248, 89th Congress, 1st Session, Committee on Interstate and Foreign Commerce, April 15, 1965, to accompany H.R. 2985: *Community Mental Health Centers Act Amendments of 1965,* (Washington, D. C.: Government Printing Office, 1965).
11. Jackson, J., "Some Issues in Evaluating Programs," *Hospital and Community Psychiatry,* 1967, 18, 23-30.
12. James, C., "Evaluation in Public Health Practice," *American Journal of Public Health,* 1962, 52, 1145-1154.

13. Joint Commission on Mental Illness and Health, *Action for Mental Health*, (New York: Science Editions, Inc., 1961).
14. Katz, M., and Lyerly, S., "Methods of Measuring Adjustment and Social Behavior in the Community: I. Rationale, Description, Discriminative Validity, and Scale Development," *Psychological Reports*, 1963, 13, 503-535.
15. Kramer, M., Pollack, E., Locke, B., and Bahn A., "National Approach to the Evaluation of Community Mental Health Programs." *American Journal of Public Health*, 1961, 51, 969-979.
16. Levy, L., Herzog, A., and Slotkin, E., "The Evaluation of Statewide Mental Health Programs," H. C. Schulberg (Chm.) Conceptual and Methodological Issues in the Evaluation of Community Mental Health Programs. Symposium presented at the annual meeting of the American Psychological Association, New York City, September, 1966.
17. MacMahon, B., Pugh, T., and Hutchison, G., "Principles in the Evaluation of Community Mental Health Programs," *American Journal of Public Health*, 1961, 51, 963-968.
18. *Mental Retardation Facilities and Community Mental Health Centers Construction Act Amendments of 1965*. Public Law 89-105, 89th Congress, (Washington, D. C.: American Psychiatric Association, 1967) 220-234.
19. *Mental Retardation Facilities and Community Mental Health Centers Construction Act Amendments of 1965: Regulations*. Public Law 89-105. Reprinted from the Federal Register, March 1, 1966.
20. *Mental Retardation Facilities and Community Mental Health Centers Construction Act of 1963*. Public Law 88-164, 88th Congress, (Washington, D. C.: Government Printing Office, 1963).
21. National Institute of Mental Health, *Evaluation In Mental Health*, Public Health Service Publication No. 413, (Washington, D. C.: Government Printing Office, 1955).
22. Novick, D., (Ed.), *Program Budgeting*. (Cambridge: Harvard University Press, 1965).
23. *Partnership for Health Amendments of 1967*, Public Law 90-174, 90th Congress, (Washington, D. C.: Government Printing Office, 1967).
24. Sata, L., Panel discussion, Russell R. Monroe, Gerald D. Klee, and Eugene B. Brody (Eds.), *Psychiatric Epidemiology and Mental Health Planning*. (Washington, D. C.: American Psychiatric Association, 1967) 220-234.
25. Smith, M., and Hobbs, N., *The Community and the Community Mental Health Center*, (Washington, D. C.: American Psychological Association, 1966).
26. Suchman, E. A., *Evaluative Research—Principles and Practices in Public Service and Social Action Programs*. (Russell Sage Foundation, New York, 1967).
27. Yolles, F., "The Role of the Psychologist in Comprehensive Mental Health Centers, The National Institute of Mental Health View," *American Psychologist*, 1966. 21, 37-41.

7: The Quest for Valid Preventive Interventions*

James G. Kelly

"One should never wear one's best trousers to go out and battle for freedom and truth."—Ibsen

Introduction

William James' legacy to psychology was remembered at the 75th anniversary meetings of the American Psychological Association in 1967 by a series of commemorative symposia focusing on humanism and the problem of will, the modern meaning of instincts, levels of awareness, and brain functions. In addition to James' substantive contributions to psychology and his eclectic and humanitarian concerns, he also began a quest for societal alternatives for social pathology that continues to speak directly to the emerging field of community psychology.

There is still much unfinished business for this legacy of William James. He challenged psychologists to create new social institutions with varied means and open ends. His own eloquence was expressed as follows:

* This chapter has benefited from the critical appraisal of Lenin A. Baler, Keith Smith, and Randolph Harper whose help is gratefully acknowledged.

"I spoke of the 'moral equivalent' of war. So far, war has been the only force that can discipline a whole community, and until an equivalent discipline is organized, I believe that war must have its way. But I have no serious doubts that the ordinary prides and shames of social man, once developed to a certain intensity, are capable of organizing such a moral equivalent as I have sketched, or some other just as effective for preserving manliness of type. It is but a question of time, of skillful propagandism, and of opinion-making man seizing historic opportunities."[13]

There are numerous current and visible illustrations of the functions of crises and social disruptions that take on the properties of miniature war-like confrontations. The wisdom of Loaste's aphorism, "In every crisis there is opportunity as well as danger," has eluded citizens, government officials and most change agents. We have failed, for the most part, to identify and moderate the social forces in our communities that are responsible for the personal and organizational casualties of change. What type of society can mobilize social change? Where in the life cycle of change programs are there opportunities to effectively influence social movements? How do interventions facilitate the evolution and development of social organizations? These searches, stimulated by William James, are still beyond the grasp of systematic knowledge.

The emergence of community psychology as a relevant area of professional engagement comes at a time when historic opportunity is seizing *us*; we certainly have not been effective in offering even miniscule suggestions for turning naturally occuring crises into social reform. While community psychologists have been active in pro-selytizing for change, we have not held positions of influence that would permit us to help identify opportunities for facilitating change, nor have we been able to pass on to others pragmatic and valid ideas that they might act upon. Eighty years after William James' words, we find that the community psychologist has joined the policy planner, the action researcher, the community developer, the urbanologist, and various groups of citizens working at making new communities. In the midst of this new and fast changing mix, we must ask: "What can we contribute that is unique?" and "How do we know that what we do counts?"

The operational issues which face community psychologists include such questions as: "When is an intervention by an outsider constructive?"; "When are interventions initiated?"; "How should interventions vary from place to place?"; "What criteria are employed to evaluate interventions?" Answers to these questions, generated out of involvement with real world affairs, suggest to the present writer that psychology must reorder its concepts for evaluating change and for conducting research, and must develop new methods of carrying out our work.

What is effective, useful and sympathetic in the design of research for univariate laboratory studies is inappropriate for the observation and evaluation of social change in natural settings and uncontrolled environments. Building towards a systematic account of the evaluation of change in social settings suggests an approach which involves multiple methods, an improvised style that emphasizes continuous participation with the local community, and a commitment to generate criteria for change. I am assuming that the community psychologist will increase his individual adaptations to social change by developing knowledge in different settings and requiring himself to create contrasting methodologies. The spirit of this personal response to the William James legacy is that adaptable knowledge will be best derived from work that emphasizes alternate methods stimulated by and appropriate to the requirements of local natural settings.

In this chapter, I will present some personal views about these issues. Three approaches to preventive interventions are described in which methods are contrasted and aims are compared. In addition, examples are offered of the type of questions that these new methods generate for verifying knowledge about personal, organizational and community change. The main thesis is that the uniqueness of community psychology is in the verification of interventions that work in a variety of social settings. If we are ingenious enough to create ways to validate these ideas, we may eventually even contribute to a redefinition of scientific activity in psychology.

Three Methods for Preventive Interventions

The following comments focus on preventive interventions that are closely identified with three types of therapeutic programs. The clinical approach which focuses upon changes in individuals or small groups can be a setting for an intervention that radiates effects that result from services offered to relevant individuals. Programs designed to initiate systematic change in an organization can also provide the setting for creating interventions that can assist an organization to deal with future crises. Community organization techniques that focus on ways to mobilize community resources for community action provide a heritage for designing preventive interventions that can enable a community to plan for its future. For each of these prototypic approaches to personal, organizational and community change, I have selected one example to illustrate the relevance of preventive programming.

For the clinical method, I have selected mental health consultation as an example of how the behavior of a consultee can be altered to affect the immediate larger environment. While most organizational change methods focus on redesigning role assignments and communication networks, altering the form of an organization also has the advantage of providing a context for developing capacities within the organization to handle future crises. The assumption is that the life style and ways of doing business of a social organization can be shifted to reduce the paralyzing features of an emergency which may face the organization. Community development is based on a dominant premise that the survival of a community depends upon its capacity to reach a new level of adaptation. Community development, with its tradition of multiple approaches and improvised formats, offers a setting for defining community change efforts which provide important guidelines for preventive intervention. In this case, the preventive intervention is developing criteria for the community to employ when setting goals for its own future.

When consultation services enable the immediate social environment to benefit from such help, this work contributes to an intervention that is preventive. If the organizational change program can rearrange the social fabric so that the new organization can deal effectively with internal and external crises, then the change program has been, by definition, a preventive intervention. Community development programs function as a preventive intervention when they enable the local community to plan for its future.

It is the present writer's view that these approaches to community change represent: (1) contrasting premises about the change process; (2) have quite different aims; (3) employ new types of data for evaluation; and, most importantly, (4) demand different principles for inferring verification of knowledge. While programs of personal and organizational change serve to generate goals that are valid as discrete accomplishments, new goals are required in order for such services to reduce expressions of maladaptive behavior. Viewing prototypic change programs as preventive interventions suggests different criteria for each evaluation. These criteria provide new options for linking change programs to social processes which may help them to become more directly related to the local host community.

Intervention I: mental health consultation as a radiating process

Descriptions of mental health consultation methods are legion, including an increasing number of efforts at evaluation that are now appearing in print (see Cowen, Gardner & Zax, 1967; and Iscoe, Pierce-Jones, Friedman & McGehearty, 1967). The work of Caplan (1964), Berlin (1962), Bindman (1959), Morse (1967), Spielberger (1967), White (1966), and others has been effective in contrasting the professional activities of a psychotherapist and a mental health consultant. All of these writings emphasize an implicit premise: the aim of the consultant is to improve the functional competence of the consultee; for example, to improve the teaching effectiveness of the classroom teacher, to assist the principal in administering his school, *etc.* The primary focus is the consultee's performance of occupational roles, and not necessarily the consultee's own personality structure or his overt expression of mental strain. The consultant's diagnostic task is to assess the consultee's competence and his ability to carry out his job in a natural setting. The assessment process differs from the diagnostic process that takes place with clients in mental health treatment facilities by including data from the immediate social environment.

The historic focus for clinical work has been the patients' or clients' feelings, perceptions and attitudes about his environment. Community mental health practice has emphasized the extension of clinical practice so that effort is expended to discuss feelings, attitudes and perceptions that relate directly to concerns about the occupational role. The type of intervention to be discussed here gives greater emphasis to clarification of how the individual copes with his environment and involves a more active, detailed exposition of the interrelationship between an individual's present behavior and his future relationships with the key persons.

If we take preventive intervention seriously, we need to derive new types of criteria for assessing its effectiveness. The payoff from a consultation program is not only an alteration in the feeling states, belief systems and aspirations of the consultee, but should also reflect a change in a person's relationships with those significant others who directly participate in his life setting. Therefore, evaluation studies should not measure changes in attitudes of consultees nor analyze samples of the interactions between the consultant and consultee, nor note changes in the consultee's self concept, for such attempts at evaluation are not congruent with a conception of consultation as a preventive intervention.

One of the early rationales for developing consultation techniques was that they allowed the professional to work with key resources in the community who in turn would have direct access to large segments of the population (Klein and Lindemann, 1961). If this rationale is taken seriously, we are faced with establishing new standards for verification. If, for example, consultation is effective in initiating a change process, then indices of effectiveness should be defined not only by changes in consultee performance, such as the classroom teacher, but by cumulative and successive changes in the behavior of significant others, for example, students in the classroom as well as the behavior of other teachers in the same school environment. The evaluation of such activities has not progressed, however, and new criteria for designing studies are in demand.

When considering research designs to document the effectiveness of consultation methods as a preventive intervention, it is essential to provide for the assessment of the radiating effects of the intervention. Since the creation of pre and post group comparisons and control groups to verify radiation effects would be prohibitive, it will be necessary to take into account what Campbell and Stanley (1963) have termed "a quasi-experimental design" in which attention is given to time and spatial effects. This type of design permits periodic measurements of selected individuals, in this case both students and classroom teachers over a period of time, before and after the introduction of an intervention such as consultation. A schema for conceiving consultation as a radiating process is illustrated in Figures 1, 2 and 3.

In Figure 1, an example is presented for two classroom teachers where one teacher is the consultee (Teacher A). This design is relevant for assessing the radiating effects of the consultation process when the consultee has frequent interactions with other persons. The elements of this design which have been diagrammed indicate that the design provides for measuring changes in the behavior of the students in each teacher's classroom. It is expected that the changes in students' behavior in Teacher A's classroom ($SI_A...SS_A$) are more salutary than those observed in the students in Teacher B's classroom. ($SI_B...SS_B$). Thus, the thesis is that an intervention such as consultation can be preventive if the consultee produces change in significant others.

Figure 1 illustrates that Teacher A, who receives consultation, is the medium for producing change in the students in her classroom.

Figure 2 diagrams a time-series design which involves repeated measurements of the students in both classrooms before and after the introduction of the intervention. Through the use of change scores and trend analysis, it should be possible to note the shifts in behavior of students in two different classrooms, one in which the teacher receives consultation, a second in which the teacher does not receive consultation. An additional feature of this design is that it permits documentation of the exact stages in the time sequence of the consultation process where its effects are seen in the behavior of students. Such work can clarify the meter of the consultation process and provide direct feedback for the practice of consultation.

Figure 1 Consultation: as a radiating process

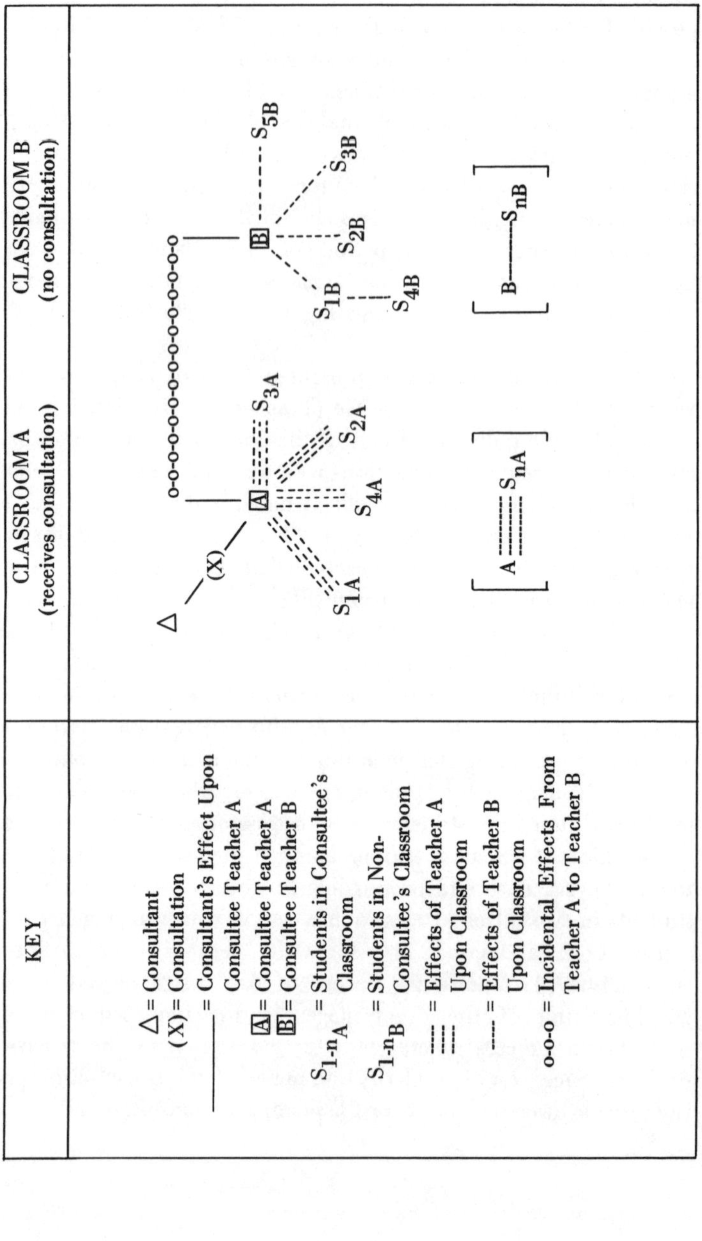
KEY
CLASSROOM A (receives consultation)
CLASSROOM B (no consultation)
Δ = Consultant
(X) = Consultation
—— = Consultant's Effect Upon Consultee Teacher A
A = Consultee Teacher A
B = Consultee Teacher B
$S_{1\text{-}n_A}$ = Students in Consultee's Classroom
$S_{1\text{-}n_B}$ = Students in Non-Consultee's Classroom
≡ = Effects of Teacher A Upon Classroom
--- = Effects of Teacher B Upon Classroom
o-o-o = Incidental Effects From Teacher A to Teacher B
S_{1A}
S_{2A}
S_{3A}
S_{4A}
S_{nA}
S_{1B}
S_{2B}
S_{3B}
S_{4B}
S_{5B}
S_{nB}

Figure 2 Consultation: as a radiating process

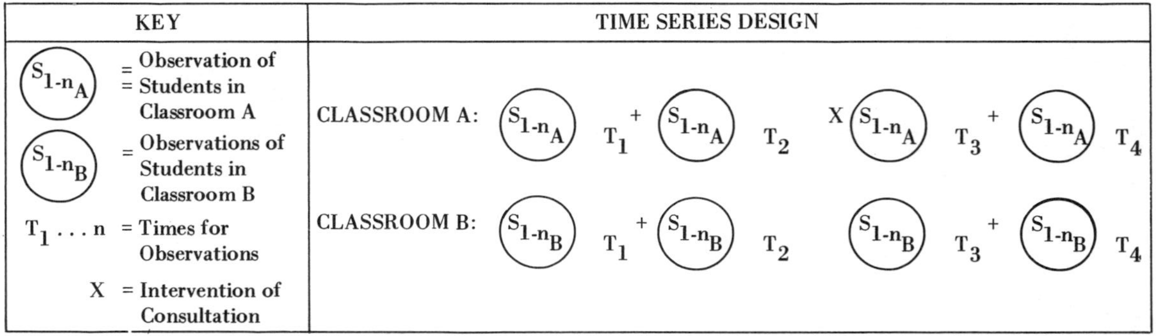

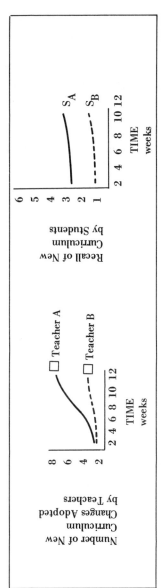

Figure 3 Consultation: as a radiating process

Figure 3 presents examples of dependent variables which reflect the effects of the consultation intervention. In the rationale for consultation previously stated, an effort is made to influence the occupational role of the consultee. Criteria for evaluating consultation as a preventive intervention can be specifically related to occupational activity such as a teacher's ability to revise her teaching methods or the quality of teacher-student interactions. In the present example, the choice was to identify the number of changes in the teaching content of the teacher. The rationale for this example is that change in the content of the curriculum is a central behavior of the teacher and defines a major segment of teaching competence. In the example, Teacher A, who received consultation, increased the number of changes in her lesson plan more than did Teacher B who did not receive this service.

The same type of predictions can also be applied to students in the classroom. If consultation has been effective as a preventive intervention, then students will be able to discriminate such effects as curriculum changes. Verification of the effectiveness of the intervention is derived from assessing changes in outcome patterns. Such quasi-experimental designs have been regarded as valid in the more successful sciences even though, as Campbell and Stanley have pointed out, they have been rarely accepted in the social sciences.

A source of uncontrolled variance that is intrinsic in this design is any unanticipated historical event which brings about a discontinuity in performance that is unrelated to one intervention. One approach to controlling this effect is to select and stratify teachers and students on the basis of the amount of contact with the consultee. As with most designs for interventions, concurrent field assessments of the local setting are also required in order to provide contextual evidence for changes in the performance of students and teachers that are inferred to be a consequence of the intervention. This type of research design reduces so-called progression effects and selection biases that often plague studies of behavior in natural settings.

With such designs, we then can test directly the effectiveness of consultation as a preventive intervention since we are no longer restricted solely to the behavior of the consultee as a criterion for outcome and can assess "fall out" effects of the consultative relationship via the performance of others in the consultee's immediate environment. This design can also include provisions for the assessment of intermediate effects, such as comparisons of consultant-consultee interactions and changes in the attitudes of a consultee regarding performance of work roles. Such observations help to establish an empirical basis for defining the process of carrying out interventions, and link outcome criteria to intermediate effects. This phase of the evaluation of intervention effects requires the identification of precise points in time where the intervention is affecting change. Suchman (1967) has an additional review of this topic in discussing outcome and process research designs.

Intervention II: organizational change as environmental restructuring

Recent work by Katz and Kahn (1966) and by Bennis (1966) presents a view of organizations, such as neighborhoods or communities, as open systems. These conceptions are based upon a premise that an organization is a series of interdependent units. Analogies have been drawn from cybernetics and general systems theory. The view of the organization is as a biological process, a view conspicuously missing in psychological treatises on organizational development. Most approaches have concentrated upon analyses in which individuals and the total organization are seen as aggregates of disconnected parts bearing little relationship to one another. The axiom of interdependent units provides a basis for a view of an organization that comes closer to the ways in which people and roles and organizational tasks are tied together under natural conditions. The behavior of people *in* organizations then is the focus of analysis in contrast to more abstract formulations of a model social structure. This point of view comes closest to an organic formulation of an organization which allows for simultaneous assessment of both organizational and personal behavior as they are portrayed through the performance of organizational roles *and* the performance of roles by individuals.

Interventions designed to affect the life of the organization can be validated via changes in the adaptive behavior of interdependent units, usually through a redefinition or realignment of various parts of the organization. If the creation of new organizational groupings, or the revision of existing social groupings, brings about overt changes in an organization's performance in coping with crises, then the intervention can be assessed by observing how the organization responds to crises. This thinking assumes that the restructuring of an organization is reflected in the total organization's ability to deal with emergencies without a significant loss of personal or operational effectiveness, and without a reduction in communication with other allied organizations.

In the same way that consultation can be used as a treatment rather than a preventive intervention, organizational change programs often deal with momentary personnel conflicts, such as, for example, issues of productivity and a variety of management-labor issues that do not involve plans for assisting the organization with long-term development. Kahn, in discussing the implications of organizational research for community mental health, commented that there have been a variety of methods to initiate change in organizations through

"various mixtures of cognitive input and peer group interaction . . . These include T-group or sensitivity training (Bradford, Bibb & Benne, 1964; Schein and Bennis, 1965); the managerial grid (Blake and Mouton, 1964; the earlier work as the Tavistock group (Jacques, 1951); and the feedback discussions in overlapping groups as developed by Mann (1957, 1964)."[15]

In commenting on these change programs, Kahn noted at least two generalizations that apply to all of these approaches; they all have been shown "to produce changes in interpersonal behavior in perceptions of self, and in attitudes toward others. Secondly, these changes are harder to produce, but more likely to endure, when they are generated in live, organizationally-embedded, ongoing groups."[15]

It is one thing to observe that an organizational change program affects the behavior of individuals in organizations, but quite a different problem to determine whether current change approaches influence the performance of individuals and organizations under conditions of stress. Still another new question is how to relate change programs to role relationships in an organization which bear directly upon the performance of the total organization in dealing with planned and unplanned change. The present writer believes that change programs which help the organization deal effectively with its future must include criteria for judging effectiveness, and must focus on additional elements of the change process. More attention must be given to changes in social influence for the help-giving behavior of persons, independent of their roles, as well as help-giving behavior that can be added to the performance of key roles within the organization. Following Katz and Kahn's formulations, such changes should substantiate precisely how the organization is interdependent. If a change effort can increase the expression of spontaneous help-giving behavior in members of the organization and create social norms so that the performance of executive functions can include help-giving behaviors, there is a possibility that there will be increased interaction and support for a wide variety of help-giving acts. The assumption is that an appropriate "organizational climate" will provide a social structure which can generate adaptive solutions for dealing with internal and external events.

The creation of an experimental design to evaluate such change programs is complex and difficult to formulate. The use of pre and post test designs and controlled measures in the study of organizations is not generally feasible since the natural life of an organization does not coincide with the aperiodic and unanticipated social events indigenous to organizations. There is one type of design, however, that may be relevant for identifying changes in the adaptive behavior of an organization. This design involves the use of similar, yet non-matched organizations, and is called, in the terminology of Campbell and Stanley, "the Nonequivalent Control Group Design."[6] For this design to be optimally effective the two organizations should be selected with attention to equivalence of their general function. This is desirable in order to provide measures to control for possible sources of "error", such as historical events affecting the organization and maturation of the organization, as well as the effects of the process evaluation. Such controls may be obtained by systematic or naturalistic observations prior to the onset of the intervention and further enhanced by continuous documentation of critical events in *both* organizations during the intervention. This operating procedure makes it possible to

122	Issues in Community Psychology

infer that any detected differences between the pre and the post tests in the adaptive behavior of the organization receiving the change program are not readily explained by the effects of extraneous variables. The possibility that differences in post intervention scores may vary directly with differences between the populations from which the selection was made can be managed by covariance analyses and other statistical techniques (Campbell & Stanley, 1963, p. 49).

The design for this type of intervention is illustrated in Figures 4, 5 and 6.

Figure 4 presents an illustration of a prototypic statement of directional influence in two organizations. At T_1, while the form of the influence varies for the two organizations, these influences are assumed to be equivalent in direction and magnitude. Following the preventive interventions, which has as its purpose the linking of directional influence, such as help-giving behavior and coping skills, organization A is expected to develop not only a quantum increase in levels of influence but also to increase the level of reciprocal influences in the organization. In sum, the aim of the intervention as a change program is to increase the interdependence of the members with each other. Figure 4 and 5 illustrate the structure of the design and the types of predictions that can be made in differentiating responses of the members of the two organizations before and after the intervention.

As an example of dependent variables that reflect an influence of the intervention, the members of organization A are expected to voluntarily devote more effort, that is man hours of work, to solve problems than the members of organization B who have not experienced such a change program. If such predictions can be made and verified, then the specific program has met the criteria of producing long-term effects for the organization as well as changes in perception, attitudes and role behaviors. The primary criterion for evaluating the change program is dependent upon identifying how *both* organizations deal with future crises. It is assumed that the organization hosting the change program will expend fewer resources, suffer fewer casualties, and revise more functions after coping with crises such as budgetary cuts, shifts in public support, or loss of decision makers, than will the "control" organization.

Figure 4 Organizational change: as a process of restructuring the environment

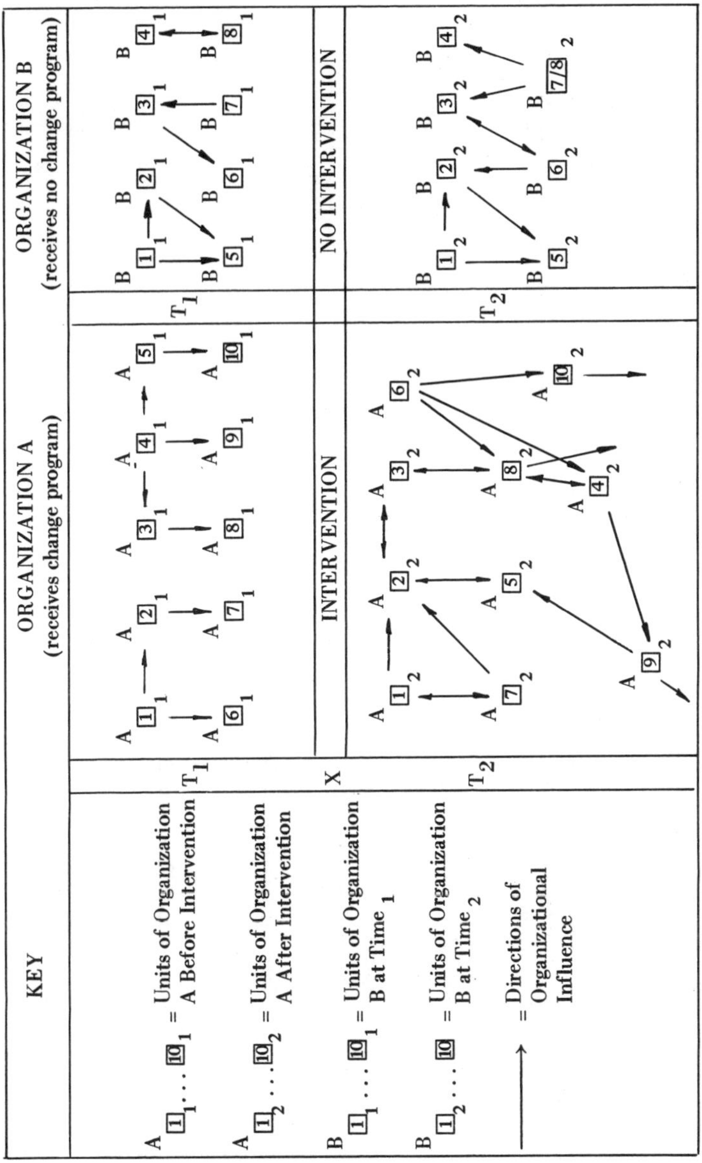

Figure 5 Organizational change: as a process of restructuring the environment

KEY	NONEQUIVALENT CONTROL GROUP DESIGN		
		ORGANIZATION A (receives change program)	ORGANIZATION B (receives no change program)

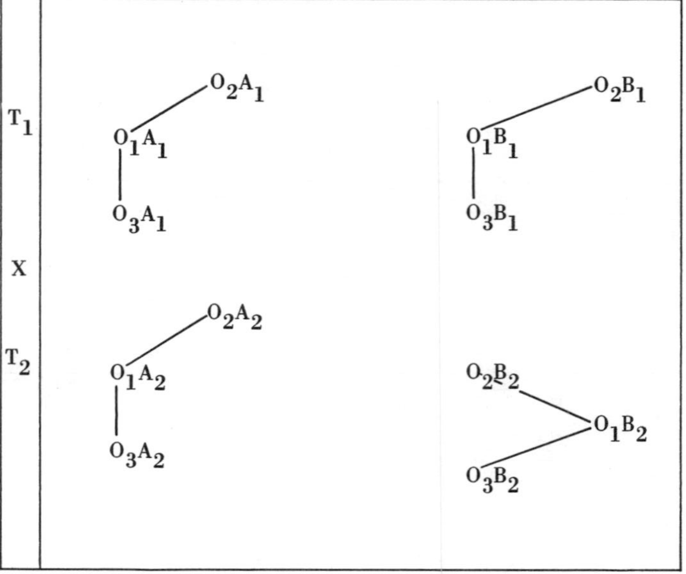

O_1A_1 = Observations (one method) of Organization A before Intervention

$O_{2,3}A_1$ = Observations (second or third method) of Organization A before Intervention

O_1A_2 = Observations (one method) of Organization A after Intervention

$O_{2,3}A_2$ = Observations (second or third method) of Organization A after Intervention

$O_{1,2,3}B_1$ = Observations (first, second or third method) of Organization B at Time 1

$O_{1,2,3}B_2$ = Observations (first, second or third method) of Organization B at Time 2

X = Intervention

T_1

O_2A_1

O_1A_1 O_3A_1

O_2B_1

O_1B_1 O_3B_1

X

T_2

O_2A_2

O_1A_2

O_3A_2

O_1B_2

O_2B_2 O_3B_2

Figure 6 Organizational change: as a process of restructuring the environment

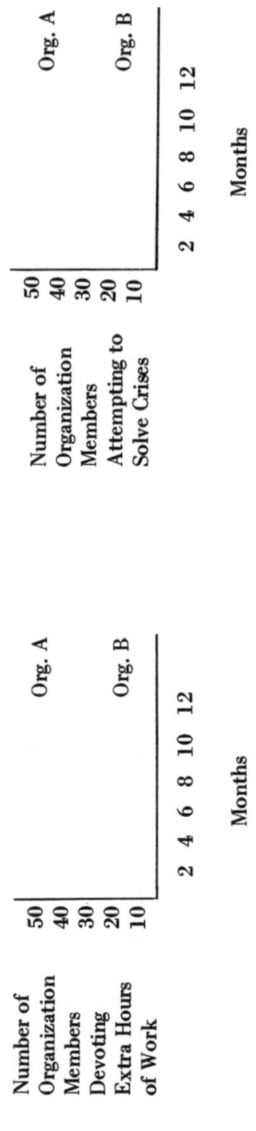

This type of design is relevant for the evaluation of community mental health programs. Many community mental health services have increased their liaison and visibility in their local communities, with the result that the public has increased demands for accountability for services, and this often poses a genuine threat to the mental health program. As a result of attempts to develop preventive programs, increasing efforts have been expended by the mental health program and citizens to create additional community resources. If organizational change programs are viewed as a lever for initiating change rearranging or redefining community services, with a decrease in specific *direct* mental health services, then an organizational change program for the community marital health center staff can be classified as preventive. Efforts at program evaluation will require coordinated and integrated studies which simultaneously assess intra-organizational activities along with morbidity rates for relevant population groupings outside the immediate organization which are directly influenced by the organization. For such community studies, the Non-Equivalent Control Group Design provides an important approach for specifying the fall out effects of interventions.

Organizational change programs with staffs of mental health programs have characteristically employed laboratory training methods (T-groups). Such programs designed as inservice training for the staff of community mental health programs often serve to realign staff resources and redistribute decision making functions regarding patient care. One potential effect of such a change program is to make it possible for the professional staff of community mental health centers working inside the center to accommodate to criteria for relevant community services developed by citizens. As roles for community mental health practice respond to change methods such as the ones described above, criteria for community mental health programs will be expected to shift and new types of data will be required for verification.

A synthesis of intervention methods can eventually bring about a greater affiliation between the clinician and the action researcher in the development of methods for assessing personal effectiveness and organizational effectiveness as reciprocal processes (Kelly 1968). Through a combined program of interventions, such as consultation and organizational change methods, interventions in a variety of settings can be more closely assessed as having positive and negative functions for the organization and for the broader community. Such interventions can describe these processes and how they mediate change, one of the most important substantive tasks for building a science of community psychology.

Intervention III: the development of a community as an evolutionary process

The previous interventions described in this chapter have been derived from contrasting premises about the change process. Consultation as a preventive intervention was viewed as a process of "radiating" change from the consultant to the consultee and to the consultee's clients. Organizational change programs were presented as examples of preventive interventions for restructuring the environment, with the goal of facilitating the organization to be more effective in dealing with crises. The third example of an intervention strategy which will now be presented is community development. This approach rests on the premise that social change is *not* a consequence of discrete man-made interventions, but rather that change occurs as a result of the evolution of the functions in a society. (Biddle & Biddle, 1968). The goal for community development is to create opportunities for a community plan for its own change. In this class of interventions, the change agent is neither a passive observer nor the final architect for plans, but a creative participant working with communities in the design and reorganization of their activities.

The term community development, like consultation and organizational change, can refer to a euphemism for Utopia or Pollyana, or it can be used to denote an ethnocentric enterprise. There are few examples to cite in which a professional change agent has been a "participant conceptualizer" in the collaborative work of a commu-

nity.†‡ More often we have been protagonists for change and have
been invested in interventions without regard for the goals of the
community. Our statements regarding community goals have been
limited to our own entrepreneurial interests. In the present writer's
opinion, until community psychology can formulate new definitions of
professional practice for community development, we will not achieve
the unfinished business which was so eloquently prescribed by William
James.

Community development is a radical departure from most professional practice in community mental health. Community development
commits the designer of an intervention to be quite clear about goals
and values he elects himself and espouses for "his" community. It is
one thing to mobilize citizens to fight for a cause; it is another to
mobilize citizens to develop plans and actions to guide their own
future. This distinction is very easy to articulate but very difficult to
translate into reality, which is the heart of the matter. Biddle and
Biddle have written at length on this theme and make the following
observation:

"Most believers in democracy have advanced to the point of admiring
controversy and stopped there. They are fighters for what they deem to
be righteous. Some have advanced further to an admiration of
compromise but the compromise they have in mind usually means a
yielding of some demands when opponents will also yield a few—a type
of horse-trading. Only a few have advanced to an appreciation of
creative reconciliation, in which new and undreamed of solutions to
problems arise out of cooperative thinking and working together. Here
is the great need and opportunity in an age of increasingly complex
problems and interdependent solutions. An encourager belongs in the
company of the creative reconcilers.

†The Phrase "participant conceptualizer" has become an apt identification for the
unique role of the community psychologist. For future archival value, this phrase
was first coined by Forrest Tyler, then of the National Institute of Mental Health,
now at the University of Maryland, in group discussions at the Boston University
Conference on Community Psychology, Swampscott, Mass., May 5, 1965.
‡‡One exception where there has been a report of a long-term collaborative work
with a community is The Cornell-Peru Project (Holmberg, & Dobyns, 1962;
Dobyns, Carlow, & Vazquez, 1962; Lasswell, 1962).

By accepting developmental goals, he does not reject political controversy. He merely leaves this necessary activity to someone else. His job is not to encourage attack upon rivals but to strengthen people's abilities to find creative solutions to conflict. He is not a political controversialist. He is a reconciler of conflict, to the end that people may become more competent to create their own solutions to problems."[4]

This quotation could be interpreted as espousing special kinds of persons who can encourage community development. The intent of the statement can also mean, however, a value to expand and diversify resources from all segments of the population. As the above comments indicate, designs for documenting this type of change program are non-existent. What little evaluation that has been accomplished is preserved in the accumulated wisdom of the change agent or in the archives of anthropological field notes.

The community psychologist has an obligation and a rare opportunity to contribute to the definition of criteria for community development. Designs for community change require momentum and the resources to sustain evaluations of the process over a long period of time. Asking any professional to think in terms of decades is unique and presents a series of taxing requirements for the research process. The dependent variables considered useful in the evaluation of consultation as a preventive intervention were the performance level of students and teachers in the classroom setting. The criteria suggested to assess organizational change were measures of coping with crises. In contrast to coping with change events, the type of dependent variables that will be required to evaluate community development are measures of *planning* for change. It is assumed that planning for change represents a higher level of organizational adaptation than either coping with crises or radiating change.

Campbell and Stanley (1963) provide a provocative initial suggestion for a design for community development known by the folksy title, "the patched-up design," or, if you prefer a more technical term, "the recurrent institutional cycle design." They describe this design as:

"a strategy for field research in which one starts with an inadquate design and then adds specific features to control one or another of the recurrent sources of invalidity. The result is often an inelegant accumulation of precautionary checks which lacks the intrinsic symmetry of the 'true' experimental designs but nonetheless approaches experimentation."[6]

In this case the research design is selected to accomodate to the unpredictable and tentative events that are generic in mobilizing citizen groups to work towards goals for achieving change at the community level. Rather than an integrated attempt to reduce sources of error, this design defines a variety of procedures to maximize opportunities for specifying the conditions under which change takes place. In this sense it is an approximation to laboratory conditions, but only an approximation. The design requires that both longitudinal and cross-section studies be continuous. It also assumes that: (1) a variety of methods will be employed; (2) the research process will be flexible in spirit; and (3) the project will be bountiful in resources so that unanticipated, spontaneous community events can be assessed.

In the same sense that consultation and organizational change programs have intrinsic validity in their own right, community development, in its aims to mobilize citizens for change, also has intrinsic merit. The thesis here is that community development becomes a preventive intervention when aroused and motivated community groups work together to effectively plan for future unknown events. This assumes that the aroused citizenry is able to utilize current resources, create new resources, and link to a maximum number of constituencies. The elements of the design are presented in Figures 7, 8 and 9.

The design combines the longitudinal and cross-sectional approaches commonly employed in developmental research. It assumes that scheduling is such that, at one and the same time, a community *in* development and a community *prior* to development can be assessed, e.g., comparisons of observations can be made at O_1 and O_2. As Figure 7 indicates, Community A, which is in the process of development, has similar planning functions to Community B early in the development cycle. The planning that is ongoing in each community is relatively

Figure 7 Community development: as an evolutionary process

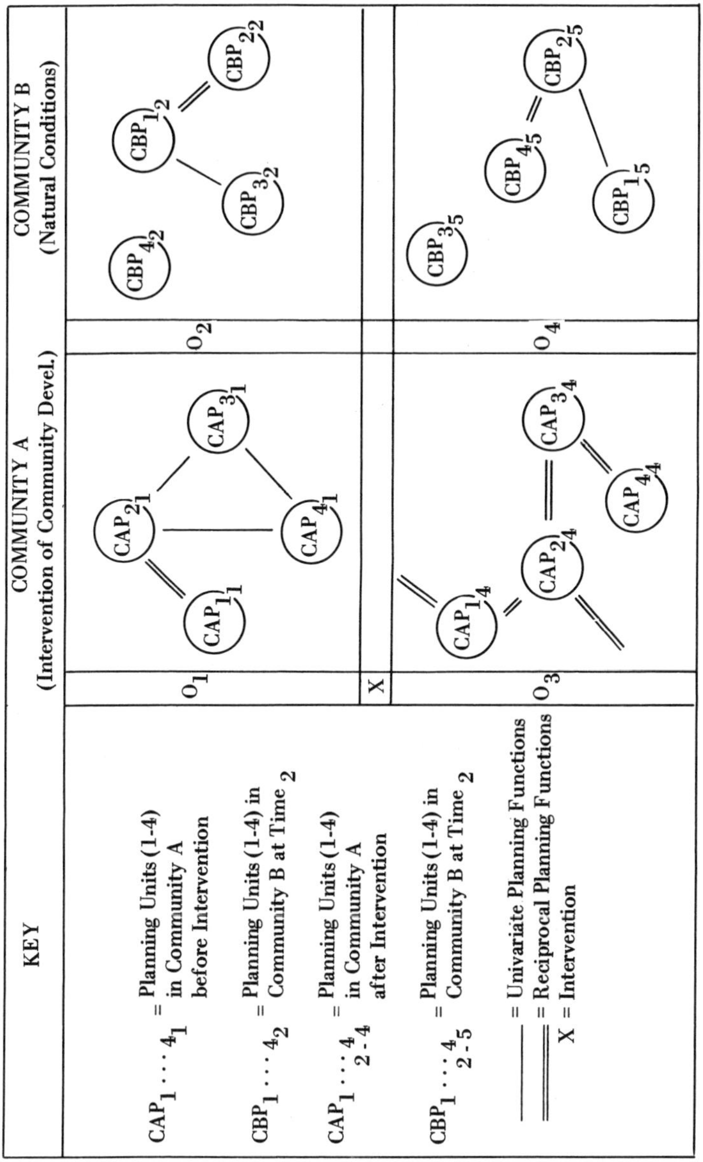
KEY
COMMUNITY A
(Intervention of Community Devel.)
COMMUNITY B
(Natural Conditions)
$CAP_{1} \cdots 4_{1}$ = Planning Units (1-4) in Community A before Intervention
$CBP_{1} \cdots 4_{2}$ = Planning Units (1-4) in Community B at Time 2
$CAP_{1} \cdots 4_{2-4}$ = Planning Units (1-4) in Community A after Intervention
$CBP_{1} \cdots 4_{2-5}$ = Planning Units (1-4) in Community B at Time 2
—— = Univariate Planning Functions
═══ = Reciprocal Planning Functions
X = Intervention
O_1
O_2
O_3
O_4
X
CAP_{1_1}
CAP_{2_1}
CAP_{3_1}
CAP_{4_1}
CBP_{4_2}
CBP_{1_2}
CBP_{3_2}
CBP_{2_2}
CAP_{1_4}
CAP_{2_4}
CAP_{3_4}
CAP_{4_4}
CBP_{3_5}
CBP_{4_5}
CBP_{2_5}
CBP_{1_5}

Figure 8 Community development: as an evolutionary process

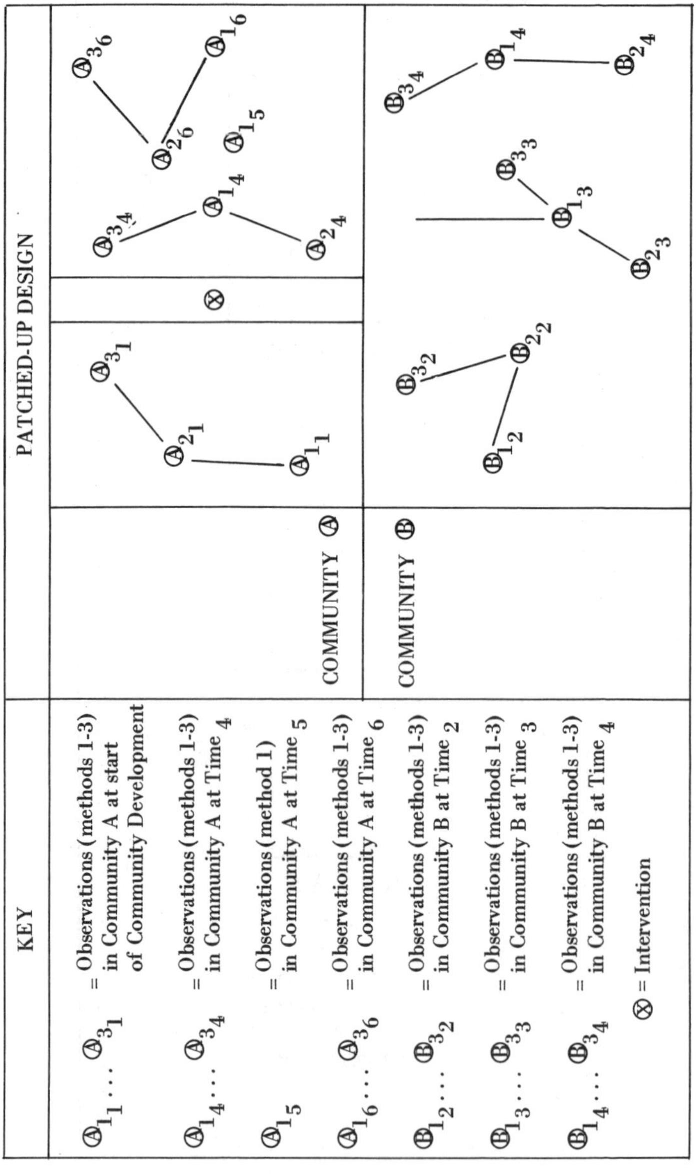

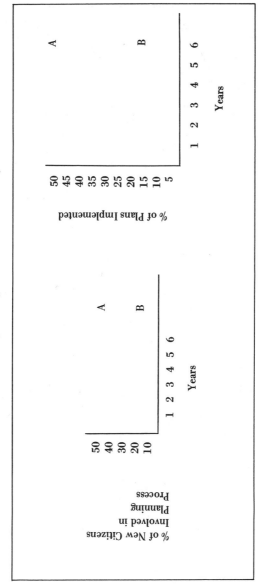

Figure 9 Community Development: As An Evolutionary Process

autonomous, largely *ad hoc*, and likely to be tied to a few individuals in formal governmental positions. Measurements in this case might be surveys, naturalistic observations, in depth interviews, participant observations, and other types of field work including attendance at formal and informal community functions. The measurements should include all that is possible and feasible in conducting a community study.

Following the community development program, observations are repeated so that a detailed evaluation of the planning process can be charted. If the program has succeeded, it would be expected that Community A will have developed more viable reciprocal planning functions, created new resources, and included more new citizens in its planning. As Figure 8 indicates, this type of design allows for taking advantage of unexpected events to document critical unplanned occurrences in the life cycle of the program, such as at time O_3, as well as comparative data collection in both communities at other times such as O_4 and O_5. Observation points can be as close as several weeks, or only six months, depending upon when the real life events take place. The total time period needed to evaluate and document the planning process per se may take several years.

Reassessing the functions of the two communities in their ability to plan for change provides a basis for many comparisons in the life of the change program. While the design does not directly control for maturation effects over time, it can be extended to assess effects over time since maturation effects can be a basic part of the study. Figure 9 presents an example of two types of predictions that can be made in assessing community development. One example is a prediction of the different number of citizens involved in working directly on the formulation and implementation of community change. Of specific interest is the proportion of new citizens who were not previously a part of the community planning effort.

The basis for this prediction is that the community development process is effective when it can continously involve, over a period of time, different citizens. The criteria refers to the number of new citizens involved who have not been involved previously in such work. The criteria also refers to increasing the proportion of persons from minority groups who are otherwise not active in the development of their local community. The effort of the community development process as a preventive intervention is to increase the diversity of citizens who are influencing change in their community.

It is expected, for example, that such an effective intervention, with its accompanying social processes, would produce a community participation curve which is S shaped. In contrast, the predicted curve for the number of persons involved and number of actions and plans implemented in control communities would not vary over time and would be only slightly positively accelerating. Such a positive acceleration is expected to reflect the effects of changes outside the community upon the local population.

Much of the emphasis in community work has been placed on the prevention of pathological conditions in individual and social settings. The prospect of obtaining knowledge about the positive development of persons in natural settings could be increased if psychologists worked to create empirical data about the ways in which communities evolve and how they establish criteria and norms. One of the important by-products of the evaluation of community development programs is the creation of a psychology of social change. How groups of persons are mobilized, how impediments to action are reduced, and how old investments of citizens are redefined and replaced by indigenous efforts are examples of discrete activities which combine to affect community goals. The evaluation of community development can also provide hypotheses about the success and failure of broader societal changes in that they provide a more restricted setting to observe the diffusion of change processes into local communities.

There is a critical need for research centers and universities to focus on the aspirations and interests of their local host communities. The contributions of the social sciences have limited relevance to understanding contemporary social problems in communities, and most public issues raise questions which go beyong the social scientists' traditional data source. We cannot expect to understand the problems of community conflict without attempting to understand the delights and the hazards of positive community change. Our present knowledge of community development comes largely from cultures beyond our own which illustrate our ideological and motivational constraints. It should be less difficult to work towards community change in the United States than in a Peruvian village, and thereby help our citizens to affect their own destiny. Community Development work is thus offered as a critical area for psychologists to offer new commitments that are expressed daily and that are lasting.

CONCLUSION

The three contrasting approaches for preventive interventions that have been described suggest new criteria for change programs. Consultation methods as a preventive intervention as presented do not focus on the symptomatic or expressive behavior of the consultee, but rather upon the radiating effects of the consultee's clients. Organizational change methods are not concerned with the productive behavior of the members of an organization, but with the members' ability to handle crises. The vertification of community development does not depend solely upon economic development, but also considers the communities competence to plan for its future. (Meier, 1965; 1966). These new criteria are required if community psychology is to contribute verifiable knowledge about the effectiveness of individuals in organizations and communities. The main thesis in these comments has been that the community psychologist views the development of knowledge as an ecological enterprise, an enterprise in which the conditions for verification are defined in terms of the specific host environment and its requirements for intervention (Barker, 1965; Kelly, 1966). A science of intervention encompasses a series of diverse and interdependent sciences, each with its unique requirements and principles for verification, and its own methods for the control of error. Psychologists can participate in this redefinition of the scientific process if we obtain for ourselves a liberal education. We can then contribute to social betterment without the hidden costs of social engineering!

Each of the three types of interventions which have been described involve unique experimental designs and methods of quality control that generate their own built-in ethics. These designs provide for the observation of naturally occurring events to help confirm or disconfirm the effects of interventions. This kind of research obviously requires a strong commitment to longitudinal studies as well as the development of research facilities that are organized to take account of unanticipated and spontaneous community events. The goals of the scientific enterprise presented have been simply stated by the philospher of science, Herbert Feigl: "Scientific explanation is where more specific or more descriptive statements are derived from general or more hypothetical assumptions."[10] The linkage between our general statements and our assumptions of the rate and direction of social change can permit the design of interventions in social settings to create a science of community psychology. For this adventure man is viewed in his natural setting, not as an atom in a smasher.

REFERENCES

1. Barker, R.G., "Explorations in Ecological Psychology," *American Psychologist*, 1965, 20, 1-14.
2. Bennis, W.G., *Changing Organizations*, (New York: McGraw-Hill, 1966).
3. Berlin, I.N., "Mental Health Consultation in Schools as a Means of Communicating Health Principles," *Journal of the American Academy of Child Psychiatry*, 1962,1, 671-679.
4. Biddle, W.W. and Biddle, L.J., *Encouraging Community Development*, (New York: Holt, Rinehart, and Winston, 1968).
5. Blake, R.R., & Mouton, J.W., *The Managerial Grid*, (Houston, Texas: Gulf, 1964).
6. Campbell, D.T. and Stanley, J.C., *Experimental and Quasi-Experimental Designs For Research*, (Chicago: Rand McNally and Company, 1966).
7. Caplan, G., *Principles of Preventive Psychiatry*, (New York: Basic Books, Inc., 1964).
8. Cowen, E.L., Gardner, E.A., and Zax, M., (Eds.), *Emergent Approaches to Mental Health Problems*, (New York: Appleton-Century-Crofts, 1967).
9. Dobyns, H.F., Carlos M.M. and Vazquez, M.C., "Summary of Technical-Organizational Progress and Reactions to it," *Human Organizations*, 1962, 21, 109-115.
10. Feigl, H., "Principles and Problems of Theory Construction in Psychology," *Current Trends in Psychological Theory*, (Pittsburgh, Pa.: University of Pittsburgh Press, 1951) pp. 179-209.

11. Holmberg, A.R. and Dobyns, H.F., "The Process of Accelerating Community Change," *Human Organizations*, 1962, 21, 107-109.

12. Iscoe, I., Pierce-Jones, J., Friedman, S.T., and McHehearty, L., "Some Strategies in Mental Health Consultation: A Brief Description of a Project and Some Preliminary Results," E.L. Cowen, E.A. Gardner, and M. Zax (Eds.), *Emergent Approaches to Mental Health Problems*, (New York: Appleton-Century-Croft, 1967) pp. 307-330.

13. James, W., from "The Moral Equivalent for War," In *Memories and Studies*, (London: Longmans, Green and Co., 1911). Also appears in *The Philosophy of William James*, (New York: The Modern Library) p. 264.

14. Jacques, E., *The Changing Culture of A Factory*, (London: Tavistock Publications, 1951).

15. Kahn, R.L., "Implications of Organizational Research for Community Mental Health," in J.W. Carter, Jr. (Ed.), *Research Contributions from Psychology to Community Mental Health*, (New York: Behavioral Publications, Inc., 1968)

16. Katz, D. and Kahn, R.L., *The Social Psychology of Organizations*. (New York: John Wiley & Sons, Inc., 1966).

17. Kelly, J.G., "Ecological Constraints on Mental Health Services," *American Psychologist*, 1966, 21, 535-539.

18. Kelly, J.G., "Toward an Ecological Conception of Preventive Interventions," in J.W. Carter, Jr. (Ed), *Research Contributions from Psychology to Community Mental Health*, (New York: Behavioral Publications, Inc., 1968).

19. Klein, D.C. and Lindemann, E., "Preventive Intervention in Family Crisis Situations," in G. Caplan (Ed.), *Prevention of Mental Disorders in Children*, (New York: Basic Books, 1961, 283-306).

20. Lasswell, H.D., "Integrating Communities into more Inclusive Systems," *Human Organizations*, 1962, 21, 116-124.

21. Mann, F.C., "Studying and Creating Change: A Means to Understanding Social Organization," in *Research in Industrial Human Relations*, Industrial Relations Research Association, No. 17, 146-167, 1957.

22. Mann, F.C., "Toward an Understanding of the Leadership Role in Formal Organizations," in R. Dubin, G. Homans, & D. Miller (Eds.), *Leadership and Productivity*, (San Francisco: Chandler, 1964).

23. Meier, R.L., *Science and Economic Development*, (Cambridge, Mass.: The M.I.T. Press, 1956).

24. Meier, R.L., *Developmental Planning*, (New York: McGraw-Hill Book Co., 1965).

25. Morse, W.C., "Enhancing the Classroom Teacher's Mental Health Function," in E.L. Cowen, E.A. Gardner and M. Zax (Eds.), *Emergent Approaches to Mental Health Problems*, (New York: Appleton-Century-Crofts, 1967, pp. 271-289).

26. Schein, E.H., and Bennis, W.G., *Personal and Organizational Change Through Group Methods,* (New York: John Wiley, 1965).
27. Spielberger, C.D., "A Mental Health Consultation Program in a Small Community with Limited Professional Mental Health Resources," in E.L. Cowen, E.A. Gardner, and M. Zax (Eds.), *Emergent Approaches to Mental Health Problems,* (New York: Appleton-Century-Crofts, 1967) pp. 214-238.
28. Suchman, E.A., *Evaluative Research,* (New York: Russel Sage Foundation, 1967).
29. White, M.A., "The Mental Health Movement and the Schools: Theory, Evidence, and Dilemma," in R.H. Ojemann (Ed.), *The School and the Community Treatment Facility in Preventive Psychiatry,* (Iowa City, Iowa: The University of Iowa Department of Publications, 1966) pp. 49-68.

8: Priorities for Psychologists in Community Mental Health

J. Glidewell

Background

In September of 1967, the Executive Committee of the Community Psychology Division (Division 27) of the APA appointed a Task Force on Community Mental Health. The Task Force was instructed to develop *cogent positions* on the *current and critical issues* confronting psychologists involved in *research* and *practice* in community mental health. The Task Force reviewed the data available about many phenomena of importance to community mental health, as well as the theories offered as interpretations of the data. The members of the Task Force held two meetings, presented one symposium, and developed a series of papers addressed to the issues identified: the conceptualization of health and disease; strategies for preventive intervention; the scientific bases for social intervention; citizen involvement in professional practice; professional influence upon public policy; evaluation of, and accountability for, professional practice; and training of professional and subprofessional practitioners. The papers are still in the editorial process; they will be submitted as a full report in the near future.

In September of 1968, the Task Force presented at the Business Meeting and submitted to the Executive Committee of Division 27 a summary report entitled, "Priorities for Psychologists in Community Mental Health." The Board returned that report to the Task Force with requests for revisions. Those revisions have been made, and this revised report is submitted to the Board for its approval and disposition.

Endorsement

The positions taken by Smith and Hobbs (1966) in their excellent statement on Community Mental Health Centers are reaffirmed here. The additional positions taken here, however, are somewhat different in that they (1) specifically apply to the work of psychologists and (2) also apply to the broad field of community mental health work, in and out of community mental health centers.

Timeliness

This report is considered especially timely for the work of the large number of psychologists now becoming deeply involved in coping with community mental health problems. As of about 1966, a majority of psychologists who were practitioners in mental health held theoretical orientations emphasizing the importance of intrapersonal phenomena (Marx, 1967). In the Chicago Metropolitan Area, for example, only about 20% engaged in any professional helping activities other than one-to-one interactions. Those who were engaged in group and community activities spent 10% or less of their time in such activities. The majority had little or no training for professional activities outside the dyadic setting (Henry *et al.*, 1967). The findings in New York and Los Angeles were similar. The data do not provide a precise assessment of it, but there has been a rapid movement of these psychologists into research and practice in community mental health, with all its emphasis on social forces, interpersonal phenomena, and preventive interventions into large social systems. Accordingly, many psychologists are being confronted with professional tasks for which neither their theory, their training, nor their experience very well equips them. It seems altogether appropriate that they should look to the professional association for considered positions on the issues they face. This report is intended to contribute to the meeting of that need to the extent that current knowledge permits. The Task Force believes that the need is urgent.

A Summary Statement of the Central Position

Psychologists involved in community mental health should place the highest priority upon collaborative, self-modifying, social interventions to prevent disorders by facilitating the accomplishment of developmental tasks, especially in children. The training and retraining of psychologists competent to perform the roles required should be assigned a top priority by the American Psychological Association.

The Promise of Preventive Social Intervention

The data concerning incidence of mental illness justify two separate conclusions with related implications. First, the data to be cited shows that early detection and treatment have not yet reduced the rate of the appearance of new cases of *infectious disorders*. Second, the data shows that, in individual human development, failures to accomplish the psycho-social tasks of one stage of development increase the vulnerability of the person to failure in accomplishing the tasks required at later stages of development. These two findings—to be elaborated and documented in the following sections—provide a basis for a shift of attention from early detection and treatment to the accomplishment of developmental tasks.

To explain this position in greater detail, it is important to review some well-known information. Methods for the evaluation of the effectiveness of psychotherapy are still developing. The criteria of effectiveness of psychotherapy have never been quite satisfactory. Even the definitions of psychotherapy vary widely and change rapidly (e.g., APA, 1967). Accordingly, any broad generalization about the effectiveness of psychotherapy lacks the specificity necessary to support a position about the allocation of resources to any particular attempt at psychotherapy. In spite of this state of affairs, it is proposed, on both scientific and humanitarian grounds, that any *reasoned and carefully observed* attempt to relieve pain and distress is a worthwhile endeavor.

In the case of the growth of the mental health movement, many failures to accomplish developmental tasks have been conceived as illnesses. In the tenor of the times, this conception had some social value. It did much to mitigate the unwise and ineffective punishment of the individual for the faults of the social systems in which he lived. It was, nevertheless, an unrealistic conception.

It was unrealistic because it implied that some healing art was required for treatment, when some ingenuity in resource allocation and training methods was really more appropriate to the problem. In addition, it was unrealistic because the resources were more often devoted to changing the individual and less often devoted to changing the social systems to accommodate to individual differences. It was unrealistic in a third way also. It applied an approach—the clinical approach—to phenomena of very high prevalence, when the approach was best suited to dealing with phenomena of very low prevalence. Historical data (e.g., Duffy, 1968) make it clear that the clinical approach has been immensely successful in curing many disorders—until the number of disorders overloads the facilities and manpower. The clinical approach did not evolve from epidemics, nor did it evolve as a socialization device for the population.

It is enough just to point to the well-known data showing how clinical facilities in mental health are now overloaded and, given current definitions of the need for treatment, are going to become more and more overloaded (Albee, 1967; Cowan and Zax, 1967). Non-clinical intervention at the system level places the responsibility for facilitating the accomplishment of developmental tasks on persons and groups more competent to discharge the responsibility—the agents of socialization. Because it is a more realistic view of the problem, it makes a more realistic use of facilities and manpower. There will remain severe failures to accomplish developmental tasks due to constitutional factors or intense stress or severe deprivation—problems of low incidence. Such problems are appropriate for treatment by clinical methods, and may be accomplished without overloading that system. (In the full report Cohen provides a conceptualization of illness and health which should relieve some of the current conflicting cliches.)

Some fifty years ago, the logic of the combination of early detection and treatment seemed particularly clear in designing the efforts to control infectious diseases. Shortening the course of the disease would necessarily reduce the number of others who would be infected. The data available, however, covering at least forty years of effort, show that the logic, however clear, did not accurately predict the findings (McGavran, 1963). Such reduction of new cases as did occur was a result of interventions into environmental systems—physical, biological, and social. The intervention was then often conceived as the sanitation of the environment, but ecologically the intervention was some sort of modification of the physical, biological, and social systems. Water purification, sewage disposal, insecticides, and even diet control and immunization—all of these were modifications of systems.

Early detection and treatment did in fact relieve much pain and distress, but it did not reduce the rate at which new cases appeared in the community. On the other hand, intervention into environmental systems did reduce the rate at which new cases appeared. If these findings can be applied to behavior disorders, the implications are clear. Intervention into environmental systems offers greater promise of prevention than does early detection and treatment. (In the full report Bloom gives an account of some approaches to preventive intervention in mental health and their epidemiological bases.)

In applying the experience from attempts to prevent infectious diseases to prevention of behavior disorders, one can cite a second set of data. Those data show that the human organism grows through a series of stages of development, each having its sequential developmental tasks—tasks quite similar for large populations of individuals. Generally, failure to accomplish the tasks at one stage influences the approach to, and limits the resources available for, accomplishing the tasks of later stages. In the positive direction, mastery of the tasks at one stage of development increases the resources for, and enhances the approaches to, the tasks of the next stage. (See the work of Hunt, 1961; B. S. Bloom, 1964; Hobbs, 1967; and LaCrosse, Kohlberg, and Ricks, in press.) Examples include the following. Training with a variety of environmental objects in everyday life at the preconceptual stages facilitates the later development of hierarchies of abstract concepts. Persons available for imitation and role-taking during early stages facilitate the movement from a reward-based conformity to an internal sense of right and wrong at the later stage. Individual differences in the developmental processes due to deprivation tend to become greater as age advances.

A third set of data shows that the accomplishment of developmental tasks is much influenced by the social systems of which the individual is a part (Hobbs, 1967; LaCrosse, Kohlberg, and Ricks, in press). Especially important are the availability, utilization, refinement, and rules of interchange of the resources in the system-resources like verbal skills, symbolic abstractions, and sense of competence as well as resources like food, clothing, and safe shelter.

The smaller systems within which the individual is in direct interaction are also much influenced by the nature of the larger systems of which they are a part. Accordingly, the accomplishment of the developmental tasks of individuals can be facilitated by modifications of larger social systems. Generally, it has been demonstrated that planned, collaborative social intervention has indeed modified individual behavior (Cartwright, 1951; M. Jones, 1953; Lewin, 1958; Lippitt, et al., 1958; Reiff and Riessman, 1965; and Loomis, 1967). It now becomes crucial to know whether a collaboratively planned intervention into a social system, with all its unanticipated consequences, will predictably and significantly facilitate individual accomplishment of specific developmental tasks. For example, will new linking social structures reduce intergroup conflict and the sense of rejection by minority-group members, as Loomis (1967) has proposed? Will an increase in the variety of functionally equivalent, active, self-selective cognitive stimuli in everyday life facilitate the development of cognitive abstraction in children, as Kohlberg (1968) has suggested? Will an increase in the turnover of a population in a community institution increase exploratory behavior and the acceptance of it, as Kelly (1967) has proposed? Will changing schools from high-density to low-density (overmanned to undermanned) facilitate the development of a sense of significance in children perceived by their peers as marginal, as Barker and Gump (1964) have proposed? It is to experimental social interventions such as these that we propose psychologists involved in community mental health should give high priority.

The Investment in Children

The idea that "the child is father to the man" is an old one. The basis for the idea lies in the knowledge about the developmental process, and knowledge about the developmental process has changed over time. It has been held that most, if not all, adult disorders are determined in the first few years of life. The data now available do not support this view (e.g., Lurie and Rosenthal, 1944; Robbins, 1966). It has also been argued that most "problem children" become mentally ill adults. This view is also at odds with current data (e.g., Stennett, 1966; Glidewell and Swallow, 1968). Much clinical attention to children has been justified as preventive of adult mental illness. This view is not supported by the data either (Levitt, 1957; Robbins, 1966; Roff, 1966). There are, however, other data.

As stated before, the data available do indicate that the human organism grows by recognizable stages of development. Failure to accomplish the developmental tasks at any one stage influences and limits the accomplishment of tasks required at later stages. Mastery of the tasks of any one stage facilitates the accomplishment of the tasks required at later stages. (See the works cited above.) These findings imply that childhood is a critical period of development, not because there is any fixation of difficulties in childhood, but because, during childhood, there remain more subsequent stages to be influenced—positively and negatively—by the accomplishment of the current developmental tasks.

Failures and masteries are cumulative and self-sustaining at increasing rates (Bloom, 1964; Hobbs, 1967). Failures at one level limit successes at the next, which in turn place even more limits on the next. Successes at one level facilitate successes at the next, which in turn provide even greater facilitation at the next. Thus, enhancement of the accomplishment of developmental tasks promotes a self-sustaining acquisition and refinement of resources—physical, motivational, emotional, intellectual, and interpersonal. The best predictor of mental health is the presence of resources, not the absence of symptoms (LaCrosse, Kohlberg, and Ricks, in press; Stringer and Glidewell, 1967).

During childhood, the individual is especially influenced by the nature of the social systems in which he finds himself—family, neighborhood, peer group, school, church (Miller and Riessman, 1961; Pettigrew, 1964; Deutsch, 1963). Accordingly, it becomes especially important to introduce new resources into those decision-making groups of adults who are particularly influential in providing and developing resources for the development of children. The family has been the traditional point of entry, but the evidence is clear that families are markedly limited by the larger systems in which they live. Greater results are more likely to accrue from collaborative experimental intervention into larger community systems. Especially important are those small groups of powerful adults whose decisions so greatly influence the allocation of community resources to families, peer groups, schools, parks, law enforcement, courts, and health services. Changes in decision-making processes in such groups have potentially very broad consequences on the human development of many people.

The Challenge of Accountability

The data available show that, as the society becomes increasingly complex and highly specialized, accountability for the consequences of social action becomes more and more vague (Haire, 1959; Indik, 1965; Berrien, 1968; Hauser, 1968; Loomis, 1967). Accompanying the increasing ambiguity of accountability, there is an increasing questioning of the good will of specialists with esoteric skills by both his clients and the community at large. As it becomes less and less possible for the client and the community to evaluate the quality of the highly specialized services received, distrust takes root and grows to cover a wider range of practitioners, from television repairmen to tax attorneys.

The data available also show that intervention into complex systems is rife with unexpected consequences. If the psychologist is to accept the obligation for accountability, the social interventions in which he is involved must be kept under constant surveillance. The unexpected consequences must be quickly known and modifications quickly made. Indeed, the goal to be pursued is that experimental social intervention can, by active feedback loops, become a self-modifying process.

Although they are not widely used, methods are available for continuing surveillance. (In the full report Kelly develops in some detail methods for the assessment of intervention.) Methods for collecting reliable and valid data are becoming more and more readily available and unobtrusive. The development of composite indices of success in accomplishing developmental tasks in whole populations is well under way. Something like a psycho-social "cost of living index" is probably feasible (e.g., see Sheldon and Moore, 1968). Research designs to provide rigorous inferences from social intervention data are already available, even if seldom employed. Media for direct, two-way communication between the public and the practitioner about data on the consequences of social intervention are widely available here and now. (In the full report, Edgerton defines the many tasks of evaluation and accountability.)

Under these conditions, psychologists involved in community affairs ought firmly to accept an old obligation and experimentally to assume a new right. Psychologists ought to accept—jointly with their community collaborators—accountability for the consequences of the social interventions in which they are involved. In the interests of science, one can expect that the store of knowledge about the nature of social systems will be significantly increased by attempts to intervene in them, if the attempts are carefully observed and clearly reported. In the interest of a realistic and just society, one can expect that clearly evaluated experiences will provide a firmer base for both a reasoned stability and a realistic social change. (See Klein, 1968.)

Such an obligation involves some new aspects of the social roles of psychologists. It involves a serious give-and-take with community agents in the design of interventions. It involves a constant surveillance over the interventions. It involves producing data that are amenable to clear-cut interpretation with respect to underlying causes and needed corrections. It also involves developing data which can be clearly understood by the community. Indeed, it involves being prepared for one's professional power, prestige, and income to be affected by the consequences of the social interventions in which one is involved. (In the full report Dörken sets out the dimensions of community collaboration in social interventions.)

Given the assumption of an obligation for accountability, the psychologist involved in community affairs may find it appropriate to begin to exercise a new right—the right to try to influence public policy. It is proposed here that a psychologist involved in community affairs ought to participate, as a part of his professional role, in the development of public policy. He ought to use the body of empirical data available to him, and he ought to make rational extrapolations from that data and his experiences to articulate clearly his views of the psychological implications of any existing or proposed public policy. (In the full report Reiff presents a more complete basis for the exercise of the right to try to influence public policy.)

In the interest of accountability, one can expect that the psychologist will find himself in direct confrontation of agents of community institutions, many of whom distrust his good will, negotiating complementary and reciprocal roles in collaborative efforts to mount self-correcting, experimental, preventive social interventions. The position is that the psychologist should give high priority to such confrontations, negotiations, and the self-correcting social interventions which can be derived from them.

Innovation in Training

The data available show that little attention is being given to training psychologists for the roles so strongly recommended here (Henry *et al.*, 1967; Marx, 1967). For some time now, the psychologist has pursued his research and practice in especially designed social systems—universities, clinics, hospitals, laboratories—systems with very little linkage with the community; social systems into which we have recommended he intervene. When he entered into collaboration, it was with others within the special system. The more he confined his work to such special social systems, the more he was rewarded by the profession in status and prestige—and sometimes in pay. Recently the direction of this trend has changed. To some extent, psychologists who collaborate with community agents and intervene into community affairs have been finding some recognition reaching them from the profession. This new trend will stimulate new programs designed to train psychologists in a science and practice of social intervention. If the estimates made here are accurate, however, it will not be necessary—at least at first—to train large numbers of psychologists to perform these roles. The proposition is that a relatively small number will meet the needs. (In the full report the issues involved in training are defined by Iscoe.)

There is another relevant set of data. The community, through its agents, has begun to intervene into the special social systems in which most psychologists work—universities, clinics, hospitals, laboratories (consult almost any newspaper). The community agents seek a greater influence over what goes on in these special systems. The psychologists may find that they are involved in collaborative social interventions with community agents whether they want to be or not. The task is to contribute to a process of reallocation of resources and power which is self-modifying in response to the consequences of each step.

Accordingly, we propose that training agencies, especially universities, but also community training agencies, give high priority to the training of psychologists competent to design, execute, and be accountable for collaborative, experimental, social intervention to facilitate the accomplishment of developmental tasks, especially in children.

Summary

Psychologists involved in community mental health should place highest priority upon collaborative, self-modifying, social interventions to facilitate the accomplishment of developmental tasks, especially of children. The training and retraining of additional psychologists especially competent to perform the roles required should be assigned a top priority by the American Psychological Association.

REFERENCES

1. Albee, G. W., "The Relation of Conceptual Models to Manpower Needs," in E. L. Cowan, E. A. Gardner, and M. Zax (Eds.), *Emergent Approaches to*

Mental Health Problems, (New York: Appleton-Century-Crofts, 1967) 63-73.

2. American Psychological Association, *Research in Psychotherapy*, (Washington: American Psychological Association, 1967) Vol. 3.

3. Barker, R. G. and Gump, P. V., *Big School, Small School*, (Stanford, California: Stanford University Press, 1964).

4. Berrien, F. K., *General and Social Systems*, (New Brunswick, New Jersey: Rutgers University Press, 1968).

5. Bloom, B. S., *Stability and Change in Human Characteristics*, (New York: Wiley, 1964).

6. Bloom, B. S., Hastings, J. T., and Madaus, G., *Formative and Summative Evaluation of Student Learning*, (New York: McGraw Hill, in press).

7. Cartwright, D., "Achieving Change in People: Some Applications of Group Dynamics Theory," *Human Relations*, 1951, 4, 381-392.

8. Cowan, E. L. and Zax, M., "The Mental Health Fields Today: Issues and Problems," In E. L. Cowan, E. A. Gardner, and M. Zax (Eds.), *Emergent Approaches to Mental Health Problems*, (New York: Appleton-Century-Crofts, 1967).

9. Deutsch, M., "The Disadvantaged Child and the Learning Process," In A. H. Passon (Ed.), *Education in Depressed Areas*, (New York: Columbia University, 1963).

10. Duffy, J., *A History of Public Health in New York City, 1625-1866*, (New York: Russell Sage, 1968).

11. Glidewell, J. C. and Swallow, C. S., "The Prevalence of Maladjustment in Elementary School Children," A report prepared for the Joint Commission on the Mental Health of Children, (Chicago: University of Chicago, 1968).

12. Haire, M., "Biological Models and Empirical Histories of the Growth of Organizations," In M. Haire (Ed.), *Modern Organizational Theory*, (New York: Wiley, 1959).

13. Hauser, P. M., "The Chaotic Society: Product of the Social Morphological Revolution," Presidential address to the American Sociological Association, Boston, Massachusetts, August 28, 1968.

14. Henry, W. E., Sims, J. H., and Spray, S. L., "Mental Health Professionals in Chicago," In American Psychological Association, *Research in Psychotherapy*, (Washington: American Psychological Association, 1967) Vol. 3.

15. Hobbs, N., "Re-education, Reality, and Community Responsibility," A paper presented at the annual meetings of the American Psychological Association. Washington, D. C., 1967.

16. Hunt, J. McV., *Intelligence and Experience*, (New York: Ronald Press, 1961).

17. Indik, B. P., "Organization Size and Member Participation: Some Empirical Tests of Alternative Explanations," *Human Relations*, 1965, 18, 339-350.

18. Jones, M., *The Therapeutic Community*, (New York: Basic Books, 1953).

19. Kelly, J. G., "The Ecology of Adaptation," Paper read at the annual meetings of the American Psychological Association. Washington, D. C., 1967.

20. Klein, D. C., *Community Dynamics and Mental Health*, (New York: Wiley, 1968).
21. Kohlberg, L., "Early Education: A Cognitive-Developmental View," *Child Development*, 1968, 39, 1013-1062.
22. LaCrosse, J., Kohlberg, L., and Ricks, D., "The Predictability of Adult Mental Health from Adulthood Behavior as Shown by Life History Research," in B. Wolman (Ed.), *Handbook of Child Clinical Psychopathology*, (New York: McGraw-Hill, in press, 1970).
23. Levitt, E. E., "The Results of Psychotherapy with Children: An Evaluation," *Journal of Consulting Psychology*, 1957, 21, 189-196.
24. Lewin, K., *Resolving Social Conflict*, (New York: Harper, 1958).
25. Lippitt, R., Watson, J., and Westley, B., *The Dynamics of Planned Change*, (New York: Harcourt, Brace, 1958).
26. Loomis, C. P., "In Praise of Conflict and its Resolution," *American Sociological Review*, 1967, 32, 875-890.
27. Lurie, L. A. and Rosenthal, F. M., "Military Adjustment of Former Problem Boys," *American Journal of Orthopsychiatry*, 1944, 14, 400-405.
28. McGavran, E. G., "Facing Reality in Public Health," In *Key Issues in the Prevention of Alcoholism*, A report of the Northeast Conference. (Harrisburg, Pennsylvania: Pennsylvania Department of Health, 1963).
29. Marx, J. H., "Therapeutic Ideologies in the Mental Health Professions," Unpublished Ph.D. dissertation, Department of Sociology, University of Chicago, 1967.
30. Miller, S. M. and Riessman, F., "The Working-class Sub-culture: A New View," *Social Problems*, 1961, 9, 86-97.
31. Pettigrew, T. E., *A Profile of the Negro American*, (Princeton, New Jersey: Van Nostrand, 1964).
32. Reiff, R. and Riessman, F., "The Indigenous Non-Professional: A Strategy of Change in Community Action and Community Mental Health Programs," *Community Mental Health Journal*, Monograph No. 1, 1965.
33. Robbins, L. N., *Deviant Children Grow Up*, (Baltimore: Williams and Wilkins, 1966).
34. Roff, M., "Childhood Social Interaction and Young Adult Psychosis," *Journal of Clinical Psychology*, 1963, 19, 152-157.
35. Sheldon, E. B. and Moore, W. E., *Indicators of Social Change*, (New York: Russell Sage, 1968).
36. Smith, M. B. and Hobbs, N., "The Community and the Community Mental Health Center," *American Psychologist*, 1966, 21, 499-509.
37. Stennett, R. G., "Emotional Handicap in the Elementary Years: Phase or Disease?" *American Journal of Orthopsychiatry*, 1966, 36, 444-449.

Index

adaptive behavior, 119
adaptive skills, 59
Albee, G. W., 25, 144
  manpower trends, 25, 144
alcoholism, 66, 75
Alcoholics Anonymous, 26
allergies, 57
Allied Health Professions, 71
American Journal of Psychology, 36
American Philosophical Association, 36
American Psychological Association, 23, 33, 35, 37, 39, 41, 52, 109, 141, 143, 151
  Community Psychology Division, (Div. 27), 141, position paper, 23
American Public Health Association, 96
  mental disorders, 96
anthropology, 42
anticipatory guidance, 5, 6
applied psychology, 38
applied science, 41
appropriations, 52
  development, 52
  research, 52
  training, 52

Bahn, A., 107
  evaluation community mental health programs, 107
Barker, R. G., 146
  education, 146
behavior, 96
behavioral disorder, 66
behaviorism, 37, 52

Bennis, W. G., 120
  changing organizations, 120
Berlin, I. N., 113
  consultation in schools, 113
Berrien, F. K., 148
  social systems, 148
biological, 56
Blake, R. R., 120
  community development, 120
Biddle, L. J., 137
Biddle, W. W., 137
  community development, 137
Bloom, B. L., 1-20, 59, 61, 73
  strategies for prevention of mental disorders, 1-20
Bloom, B. S., 145, 147
  human characteristics, 145
  student learning, 147
Board of Scientific Affairs, 52
Boulder Conference, 24
Brown, B. S., 56
  psychology and community mental health, 56
Buchner, E. F., 37
  psychological progress, 37

Campbell, D. T., 115, 118
  experimental research, 115, 118
Caplan, G., 113
  preventive psychiatry, 113
Cartwright, D., 146
  group dynamics theory, 146
Cartwright Review of World War II, 40, 42
change, 68, 136
child development, 24, 39

clinical psychology, 24, 41, 72
Cohen, L. D., 55-74
  health and disease, 55-74
Colman, D., 69
  goals and objectives, 69
community, 7, 17, 76
  clinical services, 8, 9
  health, 68, 141
  learning, 13
  mental health facilities, 23, 77
  mental health services, 78*
  planning, 50
  priorities, 11
  psychology, 24, 33, 110, 129
  social scientist, 7, 117
community intervention, 7, 53, 112,
  127, 131*-2*-3*
  citizen participation, 53
  control, 53
  development, 112, 127, 131*, 132*,
    133*, 134, 136
  organization, 112
Community Mental Health Centers
  Act, 79, 89, 90
comparative psychology, 38
Comprehensive Health Planning and
  Public Health Service Amendments of
  1966, 89
consultation, 5, 6, 23, 85, 116*, 117*,
  127, 136
Cowen, E. L., 113, 14
  emergent approaches, 113
  issues and problems, 144
crisis intervention, 5, 6, 65, 66
  initiative, 65
  self reliance, 65
criminal psychology, 39

decision making, 50
demographic studies, 16
  personal characteristics, 16

Department of Defense, 51
depression and recovery period, 38
Deutsch, M., 148
  disadvantaged child, 148
developmental behavior, 6
developmental process, 147
diagnostic testing, 24
disease, 57, 58, 64, 66
  accident, 57
  allergies, 57
  chronic, 57
  cultural view, 57
  deficiency, 57
  genetic, 57
  germ theory, 56
  heredity, 58
  immunization, 64
  internal, 58
  micro-organizm, 57
  trauma, 57
  virus, 16
direct service, 86
  early detection, 86
  habilitation, 86
  individual treatment, 86
Division of Community Psychology, 52
Domke, H., 95
  health department research, 95
Dörken, H., 75-88, 149
  community mental health services,
    75-88
drug dependency, 26
Duffy, J., 144
  public health, 144

ecological studies, 16
  environmental, 16
  neighborhood, 16
ecology of human disease, 58
Economic Opportunities Act, 79
economic status, 62

*Page numbers with an asterisk refer to illustrations or tables.

Edgerton, J. W., 89-107
  evaluation, 89-107
education, 5, 69
emergence, 24
Engel, G., 56
  health and disease, 56
environmental, 7, 25, 114
epidemiology, 13, 23
  analytic, 14
  descriptive, 14, 16
  experimental, 14
etiology, 59
evaluation, 84, 89, 92, 101
  computer, 100
  methods, 89
  resources, 93
  standards, 93
  statistics, 126
Eysenck, H., 84

Feigl, H., 137
  theory construction, 137
field research, 82
  operational research, 82
  problem identity, 82
  staff development, 78
Fiessman, F., 148
  subculture, 148
Freeman, H., 94
  intervention programs, 94
Friedman, S. T., 138
Fuller, B., 36, 42
  ideas and integrities, 36, 42
Fuchs, V. R., 69, 70
  medical costs, 69, 70

Gardner, E. A., 65, 113
Gauzer, U. J., 70
  medical model, 70
Glidewell, J., 95, 141-153
  priorities for psychologists in com-
    munity mental health, 141-153
  health department research, 95

maladjusted children, 147
Goffman, I., 79
Gordon, I., 65
  education, 65
Greving, F. T., 94
  evaluation community, 94
Gump, P. V., 146

Hagerty, G., 106
  community mental health program,
    106
Haire, M., 148
  organizational growth, 148
Hall, G. S., 43, 44
Hauser, P. M., 148
  chaotic society, 148
Headstart, 65
health, 55, 62, 69, 70, 71
  future, 70
  medical, 70
  present, 70
  psychological, 70
  services, 71
Henry, W. C., 142, 150
  professionals, 142
Herzog, A., 107
  evaluation statewide, 107
Hilleboe, H. E., 68
  manpower health, 68
Hobbs, N., 92, 145
  community mental health centers,
    142
  re-education reality and community
    responsibility, 145
Hughes, C. C., 69
  health and change, 69
human welfare, 63
Hunt, J. McV., 145
  intelligence and experience, 145
Hutchison, G., 94
  evaluation, 107

Indik, B. P., 148
individual, 4, 17

characteristics, 17
industrial psychology, 39
infectious disease, 143
institutions, 52, 64
interpersonal phenomena, 142
intervention, 4, 7, 73, 76, 95, 104,
    111, 151
  anticipatory guidance, 5
  biological, 66
  community, 7
  consultation, 5, 113
  ecological models, 95
  environmental, 99
  epidemiological, 95
  identifying crisis, 5
  physical, 145
  professional, 49
  psychological, 5
  social, 66, 145, 149, 151
  systems analysis, 95
Iscoe, I., 21-32, 138
  professional and subprofessional
      training, 21-32
  mental health consultation, 138

Jackson, J., 93
  evaluation, 93
Jacques, E., 120
  changing culture, 120
James, G., 93
  evaluation public health, 93
James, W., 109
  moral equivalent for war, 109
Joint Commission on Mental Illness
    and Health, 91, 102
Jones, M., 146
  therapeutic community, 146
Journal of Abnormal and Social
    Psychology, 39

Kahn, R. L., 119, 120
  organizational research, 120
  social psychology of organizations,
      119

Katz, D., 119
  social psychology of organizations,
      119
Katz, M., 106, 107
  community mental health program,
      106
  measuring adjustment and social be-
      havior, 107
Kelly, J. G., 109-139, 146
  adaptation, 146
  preventive intervention, 109-139
Klein, D. C., 114, 149
  community dynamics, 149
  preventive intervention, 114
Kohlberg, L., 145, 146, 147
  adult mental health, 145, 146, 147
  education, 146
Kramer, M., 107
  evaluation community mental health
      programs, 107

LaCross, J., 145, 146, 147
  adult mental health, 145, 146, 147
Lemkau, P., 8
Levy, L., 107
  evaluation statewide, 107
Lewin, K., 146
  social conflict, 146
Lewin's theories, 40
Levitt, E. E., 147
  child psychotherapy, 147
Lindemann, E., 114
  preventive intervention, 104
Lippitt, R., 146
  planned change, 146
Locke, R., 107
Loomis, C. P., 146
  conflict, 146, 148
Lowery, H., 106
Lurie, L. A., 147
  problem children, 147
Lyerly, S., 107
  measuring adjustment and social
      behavior, 107

MacMahon, B., 94
  evaluation, 107
maladaptation, 73
maladjustment, 58
management, 64
manpower development, 30
Marx, J. H., 142, 150
  therapeutic ideologies, 142, 150
Mase, 71
Meier, R. L., 136
  developmental planning, 136
mental disorder, 1, 76
Mental Health Facilities Act, 23
Mental Health Manpower Study, 22
mental health services, 75
Mental Health Studies Act of 1955, 22
McGauran, E. G., 145
  public health, 145
McHehearty, L., 138
Miller, G. A., 63
  human welfare, 63
Miller, S. M., 148
  subculture, 148
Montefiore Hospital, 86
morale, 40
Morse, W. C., 113
  classroom teacher, 113
Mouton, J. W., 120
  community development, 120

narcotic, 26
National Advisory Council on Radio
  and Education, 39
National Commission on Community
  Health Service, 71
National Institute Mental Health, 93
National Research Council, 39
  Advisory Committee on Personnel
    Problems, 39
  Emergency Committee in Psy-
    chology, 39
  needs, 10, 31
    human, 10, 31
Non-Equivalent Control Group Design,
  126
nonprofessional sector, 21, 26
normative crisis, 5, 6
Novick, D., 105
  program budgeting, 105

organizational change process, 122,
  123*, 124*, 125*
organized psychology, 35, 36, 42, 45,
  51
  guidelines, 51
  internal crisis, 51
  war and military, 51

participant conceptualizer, 128
Partnership for Health Admendment of
  1967,
Peach Corp., 82
personality, 39
personnel problems, 41
  psychiatric, 41
  rehabilitation, 41
Pettigrew, T. E., 148
  negro american, 148
philosophy, 36
Pierce-Jones, J., 138
political science, 50
Pollack, E., 107
Poverty Movement, 79
prevention, strategies for, mental disorders, 1-20
preventive intervention, 109, 114, 135,
  142
primary prevention, 1, 3, 13, 18, 76
  analytic, 13
  consultation, 114
  disease, 62
  education, 62
  environmental control, 62
  epidemiology, 13, 23
  experimental, 13
  mental disorders, 75
  prevention issues, 2
  research, 2

strategies, 2
priorities, 52, 141
problem children, 147
professionals, 9, 11, 21, 29, 35, 71, 72,
    77, 103, 141
  clinical psychologist, 103
  evaluation, 97
  guidance, 69
  psychologist, 29, 72
program development, 83, 84
  need survey, 83
  resource development program, 83,
    84
program evaluation, 92, 98
promoting human welfare, 51
Psychological Bulletin, 36
psychological disorder, 55
Psychological Review, 36
psychological warfare, 40
psychology, 38
  comparative, 38
  experimental, 38
psychopathology, 25
psychotherapy, 24
physiology, 36
public policy, 33-54
public welfare, 52
Pugh, T., 94
  evaluation, 107

Ricks, D., 145, 146, 147
  adult mental health, 145, 146, 147
Rosenthal, F. M., 147
  problem children, 147

Sarason, I., 70
  medical model, 70
Sata, L., 104
  epidemiology and mental health
    planning, 104
Schaeffer, M., 68
  manpower health, 68
sensivity training, 120

Sherwood, C., 94
services, 70, 75
Sigerist, H., 56, 60, 61
  civilization, 60, 61
  disease, 60, 61
Slotkin, E., 107
  evaluation statewide, 107
Smith, M. D., 142
  community mental health centers,
    142
social action, 148
  accountability, 148
social agencies, 70, 76
social change, 111
  community, 111
  organizational, 111
  personal, 111
social conditions, 35, 67, 110
  advance knowledge, 110
  existing knowledge, 110
social context, 46, 47
social crisis, 33, 36, 52, 110
social forces, 142
social issues, 52
social needs, 26, 70, 72
social organization, 60
social pathology, 25
social policy, 50
social problems, 33, 47, 64, 90
  civil disorder, 33
  correcting causes, 64
  failure of responsibility, 33
  professional and nonprofessional, 64
  racial conflict, 33
  war, 33
social psychology, 39, 40, 41
social reform, 53
  civil rights, 53
  war on poverty, 53
social science, 52
social scientist, 17, 34
  community leader, 34
  public educator, 34

social engineer, 34
social systems, 73
Society for the Psychological Study of
  Social Issues, 43
sociocultural, 59
sociology, 42, 50
Spielberger, C. C., 113
  community consultation, 113
Sprigle, 65
strategy, 61, 75
Stainbrook, E., 56, 59
  health and disease, 56, 59
stress, 57, 65
Suchman, E. A., 119
  evaluative research, 119
Swallow, C. S., 147
  maladjusted children, 147
Swampscott Conference, 24
systems analysis, 105
systems resources, 146
systems theory, 119

Task Force, 141
testing, 38, 39
therapeutic programs, 112
trained manpower, 28
training, professional and subprofessional, 21-32, 77, 150
  behavior modification, 28
  career orientation, 78
  personnel, 79
  perspectives, 29
  sources, 28
  staff development, 78
  technicians, 28
training programs, 24

training skills, 80
  sensitivity, 120
treatment, 66, 75
  economic insecurity, 75
  health services, 67
  homes, 75
  ignorance, 75
  organized services, 66
  problems of living, 69
  social alienation, 75
  working conditions, 75

underlying difficulty, 55, 56
  professional, 55
  treatment, 55

value judgment, 48
Van De Rict, E., 65
Vista, 82

War Production Board, 42
  Office of civilian requirements, 42
White, M. A., 113
  schools, 113
WICHE, 81
World War I, 37, 41
World War II 24, 25, 39, 41, 62

Yerkes, R. M., 37
  psychology and national service, 37
Yolles, F., 102
  psychologist in comprehensive men-
    tal health center, 102

Zax, M., 113, 144